Parenting Children
With Disabilities

PEDIATRIC HABILITATION

series editor   ALFRED L. SCHERZER

Cornell University Medical Center
New York, New York

AN IMPORTANT MESSAGE TO READERS

A Marcel Dekker, Inc., Facsimile Edition contains the identical content of the original MDI publication.

Reprinting scholarly works in an economical format ensures that they will remain accessible. This contemporary printing process allows us to meet the demand for limited quantities of books that would otherwise go out of print.

We are pleased to offer this specialized service to our readers in the academic and scientific communities.

Parenting Children With Disabilities

A Professional Source for Physicians and Guide for Parents

PEGGY MULLER MIEZIO

MARCEL DEKKER, INC.   New York and Basel

Library of Congress Cataloging in Publication Data

Miezio, Peggy Muller, [date]
   Parenting children with disabilities.

   (Pediatric habilitation ; v. 4)
   Bibliography: p.
   Includes index.
   1. Handicapped children—Family relationships.
2. Parenting. 3. Child development. 4. Physician and
patient. I. Title. II. Series. [DNLM: 1. Child,
Exceptional. 2. Handicapped. 3. Parent-child relations.
W1 PE 167K v. 4 / WS 105.5.H2 M632p]
HQ773.6.M52   1983   649'.15   83-6604
ISBN 0-8247-1090-8

MARCEL DEKKER, INC.

270 Madison Avenue, New York, New York 10016

Current printing (last digit):
10 9 8 7 6 5 4 3

PRINTED IN THE UNITED STATES OF AMERICA

FOREWORD

A virtual revolution in medical technology over the past decade has
had an enormous impact upon pregnancy and the developing child.
New techniques now result in problem pregnancies being sustained and
deal effectively with the difficult labor or delivery. Rational decisions
based upon predictable laboratory data enable determination as to
whether the fetus is best nurtured within the natural environment of
the mother's uterus or in the scientifically duplicated environment of
the neonatal intensive care center. Perinatology has made the "delivery" of the most viable infant possible for further newborn care. Infants are surviving today who virtually had no chance 5 years ago.
Many may have evidence of structural malformations and neurologic
or developmental abnormality.

In utero diagnosis has expanded its horizons from determining
sex and chromosomal abnormalities to identification of structural
malformations and metabolic disorders. The choice of continuing a
pregnancy is clearly within the grasp of both parent and professional.

Early identification of abnormal structure and development in
the very young infant is an increasingly more sophisticated process.
It is being demanded professionally as an outgrowth of the technologies
that affect survival.

A final logical step in the sequence of this revolution in early
care is the provision of programs to assist parents in care and management. An array of treatment programs involving physical, occupational,
and speech therapies are becoming widely available. Often these are
combined with infant educational programs to provide a "meducational"
approach to involved infants.

At the same time, multidisciplinary medical care; therapy activities; and educational, psychological, and social service programs are increasing at various levels under the auspices of both voluntary and governmental agencies. Such programs are now designed for a wide spectrum of people from young infants through the ever-increasing numbers of surviving adolescents and young adults. They are having a major impact on functional development and management needs for all degrees of severity of developmental disability.

Today's physician is increasingly touched by these developments at every stage. Technological training generally enables appropriate understanding of and communication with the concerns of a "risky" pregnancy or delivery; the factors to be considered in prenatal diagnosis; and the procedures necessary for survival in intensive neonatal care.

On the other hand, variable knowledge exists concerning how the physician communicates the initial and subsequent information to parents about the diagnosis or medical problem. This is equally true with professional referrals for further diagnosis, workup, or therapy.

The needs and problems of the surviving child and his or her parents are often considered out of professional bounds by the physician. Frequently there is limited insight into the needs for medical guidance and direction in the whole array of concerns which are the legacy of the involved child and family. These range from identifying appropriate agencies for help, through dealing with developmental problems, effects of family and environment, to social and financial issues.

The physician or other health-related professional who deals with such children and their families has no choice but to become involved and at a level of appropriate professional competence. This means that there must be comprehensive awareness of needs and concerns of both parent and child as they grow.

Up to the present there have been relatively few written materials dealing with the issues involved in the growing handicapped child and his or her family. The present volume will help to correct this deficit. It has two major thrusts. The first is directed to the professional, to create an awareness of the issues involved and to help him or her obtain an insight into ways of building professional direction in the course of clinical contact with the family. To anticipate need is the first step in helping to reduce many of the problems that can greatly limit development.

The second target of this volume is the affected family itself which often needs guidance and direction into anticipated areas of concern. The family can be assisted in seeking appropriate sources of professional help, financial and other practical considerations, and working in a stepwise fashion on relevant priorities at each level of development.

Professionals and parents need this source to communicate better and to work toward achieving the maximum functional potential of the child. It is essential that the physician in particular refer parents to a book of this kind early in their relationship. The professional must be aware of the many facets of impact on the family and be available for support, guidance, and management at the earliest possible time. The needed areas of professional follow up include problems in growth and development, appropriate therapy or treatment, school, and vocational concerns.

It is anticipated that this work will become a major tool in the hands of professionals for their own background information. At the same time, it should be a primary reference source suggested to parents as early as possible so that they can plan intelligently for the special needs of the affected handicapped child.

Alfred L. Scherzer, Ed.D., M.D.
Clinical Professor of Pediatrics
Cornell University Medical College

PREFACE

This is a book about parenting the child with a disability. It is
about the issues that must be confronted and resolved, but it is
also about the pain, the fears, and the joys of this experience. It is a
distillation of personal and professional experience. I am the parent of
of a child, now a teenager, with a disability. But this is not our personal
story. It represents almost 20 years of experience as a nurse, a social
worker, and a leader in a national voluntary organization.

Most people in today's world who become parents choose to do
so. No one, however, wishes that the child should be born with a
disability. The news is always unwelcome, unexpected, unwanted.

All aspects of a family's life are affected. The prospect of raising
this child looms as a task of monumental demands and responsibilities.
All the family's decisions — where it lives, how it lives, and what it
does — must now be made with the child's needs in mind. The implications of the disability may range from the smallest details of daily
living, such as how the furniture in the house is arranged, to ultimate
questions of independence and quality of life for the child as an adult.

Basic life goals, values, and beliefs of parents are shaken and
tested. Some will be strengthened, while others will be found wanting
and will be discarded. If this book can be said to have a philosophical
point of view, it is that of the interrelationships of our personal, family,
and social systems. The individual parent's response is intricately
enmeshed with the responses of the child, the spouse, other family
members and friends, and the professional people who become involved. So too is the family's experience interwoven with the society
at large: its values, its attitudes, and its acceptance or nonacceptance
of persons with differences.

How are ordinary people, caught unprepared, to incorporate this "disaster" into their lives? Resolve the issues involved? Live with pain and uncertainty? Build an altered life? Find joy? Many of them are, quietly, day by day, successfully managing these difficult questions.

It is the goal of this book that an examination of the issues involved can help the process of understanding and growth for parents, physicians, and other professionals who wish to help them. It is designed to provide for parents a sharing of experiences as well as suggestions for ways to deal with problems and places to turn to for help. For those in the helping professions, its intent is to offer an understanding of the parental experience and to suggest possibilities for intervention and assistance.

Most of the major issues facing parents are similar regardless of the nature of the disability, be it physical or mental. Likewise, the severity of the disability, within very broad parameters, has little to do with the experience of confronting these issues. A family whose child has a disability which an outsider may consider as "mild" may well have as much or as little difficulty as a family whose child is objectively more severely affected. Exceptions, of course, are the child who is not expected to progress beyond the level of infancy or for whom death is anticipated.

The book's primary organization is divided into major stages of the developmental life of the child. Thus, after the sections on acceptance and the impact on the family will be found sections on the issues of early childhood, middle childhood, and adolescence. Interspersed with these are chapters on issues that tend to have implications and repercussions extending beyond these divisions, such as finding and utilizing professional assistance, learning the advocacy role, and financial concerns. Many chapters will conclude with a series of questions designed to assist parents as they think about how these issues relate to their own lives and experiences.

The use of pronouns (he or she, him or her) has been somewhat of a dilemma for me. I am sensitive to the subtle effects of continued use of masculine pronouns, but at the same time I find that to use both "he or she" or "his or her" at all times is clumsy and distracting. For this reason, some of the chapters of this book contain masculine pronouns while others use the feminine versions. While this is not, to my mind, an entirely satisfactory solution, it is at least *a* solution.

I owe a debt of gratitude to the many individuals with disabilities and parents who have educated me and expanded my understanding of the many issues involved. My own life has certainly been enriched for having met and shared with them. I would also like to thank Dr. Alfred Scherzer for his painstaking review of this manuscript and his encouragement. My family, including my daughters Karen and Dana, deserve thanks not only for their patience and support, but for what they have taught me about living.

Peggy Muller Miezio

CONTENTS

1
ISSUES OF ACCEPTANCE

"There is something wrong with this child." The words have a reality that cannot be denied. They may be spoken, gently or harshly, by a white-coated figure who suddenly becomes nameless and faceless to the parent who stands alone. Only the words echo in the parent's mind: "There is something wrong with this child."

The figure in the white coat may continue to speak, but the parent cannot hear. The parent, in shock, is struggling to think the unthinkable. It is impossible, at such a moment, to comprehend the meaning of the words being spoken. It is not even possible to formulate or to ask questions about them.

Or the words may rise, unbidden, in the thoughts of a parent. The parents have taken the newborn child home to love, expecting the usual colic and diapers and pleasures. They have tried not to notice as the expected milestones of infant progress have arrived, and passed, without change. Icy tentacles of fear have begun to pierce their consciousness. "No," they think, "I cannot speak of this fear or even think of it. It cannot be real. If I say the words out loud, even to my spouse, it might become real, so I will remain silent." But the thoughts persist, until finally they must be given words. "There is something wrong with this child."

Does it make a difference how the discovery happens? The parent who receives the news in the delivery room has little room to maneuver; the condition is present, it is real, and it is inescapable. The parent who first notices lags in development at home, on the other hand, may undergo a long period of uncertainty with emotionally draining alternations of hopes, fears, and despair. This parent no longer knows which is the reality, the hopes, or the fears. This roller coaster of

uncertainty may continue for years. Barsch[1] reports that his data
suggest that parents are aware of deviance from expected developmental patterns for from 1 to 4 years before a definitive diagnosis is
reached. In other work, Meadows found that one-third of the parents
of children who were deaf in her study had the first doctor they
consulted deny the suspected deafness existed. Sixty percent of these
parents had to consult four or more doctors before an accurate
diagnosis of the child's problem was made.[2]

However, the crux of the matter is the fact of the happening,
not the manner of its happening. The concerns of raising a child with
a handicap are much the same regardless of how that handicap is
discovered. Likewise, there are more similarities than differences in
the experience of becoming the parent of a child with a problem, be
that problem physical, mental, or emotional.

What has happened to each of these families is that the entire
world has changed; and it will never be quite the same again. Dreams
have been abruptly, or slowly, shattered. As the moment of initial
shock passes and the parents are able to begin to grasp some of the
implications of this event, they peer into a very long and very dark
tunnel. Grief and dismay accompany the realization that the child's
disability is permanent. The prospect of the future seems to offer
no escape, no respite from this immovable reality. The parent realizes
that all the rest of his or her own life will be colored by the fact of
the disability.

To the new parent, it all seems quite overwhelming. But many,
many families will proceed to incorporate this new situation into
their lives. They will love their children and enjoy the abilities and
accomplishments the child does have. They will seek out proper
treatment for their children and provide support and assistance for
them during the process. Values and goals held by the parents will be
weighed and reexamined. As pain and disappointment become part
of life experiences for families, new perspectives on which things are
important and which are unimportant may emerge. Much human
growth is possible as families realize that while life may be different,
it is not over. Laughter and joy can again take their places in the
family's experiences.

This process does not take place all at once. It evolves slowly,
amid the constantly shifting mosaic of the child's growth, the
development of the other members of the family, and the nature of
the interactions between themselves and the many segments of the
larger world in which they live.

Describing what happens to families, and how they cope, has
two pitfalls. The pain and stress of a child's disability and the
demands it places on a family are real. Detailing how this affects the

members of a family and the relationships within a family seems unsatisfactory because it tends to leave readers with an impression of unending gloom and tragedy. The picture seems unbalanced. To speak of the ways in which families succeed, however, is to run the risk of sounding simplistic. "Success," in this situation, includes pain and struggle, and it is both dishonest and unjust to minimize these. Parents of children with disabilities are not "special people" who have been singled out because they can be heroic and can triumph over adversity. We know that some families cannot. Specialized programs to facilitate the adoption of children with disabilities are appearing to help find alternative homes for children who need them. Families with a disabled child, like all families, are continually growing and changing. The family of a disabled 5-year-old may sound like quite a different family if they are interviewed again when that child is 15 years old.

Key points and issues that arise during the course of this evolution can be identified. Families will, of course, differ very widely in the degree of ease with which they negotiate each of these issues. Some may become "stuck," and need help in discovering alternative ways of handling the problems. An understanding of the issues commonly faced can help the parent to be better prepared and to feel less alone, and can suggest for the professional possibilities for intervention and assistance in the process.

Much has been written about the need for parents to accept their child's disability. Certainly, to continue to wage furious battle with what cannot be changed is draining and unproductive. The disability has happened. In most cases, it can be ameliorated but not undone.

Nevertheless, there are some problems with our notions of what constitutes acceptance and our ideas of whether a particular parent has "accepted" the child's disability or not.

We may have unrealistic ideas about the meaning of acceptance. As Roos points out in relation to retardation, it may be too much to ask to expect parents to accept this with equanimity. Our society places too much value on intelligence for this to be possible.[3] The very high values our culture places on youth, slimness, mobility, and physical beauty may make this kind of acceptance almost as difficult for a physical handicap.

We tend to speak of acceptance as though it were all or nothing; as if it were either accomplished or not accomplished, and once done, done forever. Brown and Moersch, along with others, urge us to "abandon simplistic and static concepts of parent acceptance"[4] since all parents both accept and reject a child at different times.

Acceptance of a disability in the context of our society is a multifaceted phenomenon. One's evaluation of acceptance will depend on which aspect of the complex mosaic one is looking at, and at what time. The demands and implications of a disability will change over time with the development of the child and the environment of the society and its attitudes, values, and opportunities for her.

The experience of preparing for the birth of a child ordinarily encompasses a great deal of planning. Many dreams and fantasies are woven around the prospect of a totally fresh start for a human being. Often, the unfulfilled and even unrecognized hopes and aspirations of the prospective parent make up the fabric of the possibilities and potentials for the yet unborn child.

Few children, of course, ever grow up to fulfill the idealized dreams of expectant parents. Most parents, however, have many years to get to know and adapt to their children as they really are with all their own strengths, weaknesses, and human foibles. Even as the child proves not to be possessed of the great beauty, talent, or outgoing personality of the parent's fantasies, other more real skills and strengths are gradually emerging. The parent learns to find joy in the talents and abilities the child does have.

This process of putting aside the previous fantasy for the present reality ordinarily proceeds slowly and gradually enough to be all but unnoticeable. This is not so for the parent who must stand and look at her infant in the newborn nursery and know that this child must begin life with something less than the babies who lie squalling around her. The pain of knowing that those dreams are not to be is acute and devastating.

Parents who come to this experience are all unprepared. They may, however, have little else in common. They may be young or old, have many years of education or only a few, be financially comfortable or struggling to make ends meet; their marriages may be satisfying or in trouble or they may not be married at all.

We are all the products of our families and our culture as well as of our own natures. Ideas and attitudes about differences or disabilities are a part of each of us, whether we are aware of their nature and origins or not. Our images and perceptions may stem from dim childhood memories of hushed talk of "monstrosities," "cripples," or "idiocy" or from televised appeals to feel pity or guilt long enough to write out a check and drop it in the mail. The fortunate among us have had the experience of knowing a real person living a satisfying life with a disability.

It is important to recognize that this is just as true for the professional person in the situation as it is for the parent, and that what happens between them in their interactions will be influenced by the attitudes and reactions of both.

The professional person who must deliver the bad news to the parent may have a difficult time. He or she may experience feelings and reactions that may be as intense as they are unexpected. Feelings of helplessness, sorrow, and even guilty relief that it has happened to someone else are common. The situation is a painful reminder of human vulnerability and of the professional's own limitations.

Knowing what to expect — that reactions of shock, denial, anger, and grief are natural and normal — can help somewhat, but the position of deliverer of bad news remains a painful and uncomfortable one. One can only soften the edges a bit; the impact of the blow remains. It may help to recognize that one may bear the brunt of parental anger simply because the anger is so overwhelming that it needs an outlet, and that as the bearer of bad tidings one just happens to be a reachable target.

Nevertheless, some key elements which will help to meet parental needs as the news is delivered can be identified. What kinds of things do parents need when they are being told of their child's problem?

The truth, of course, must be told. It cannot be avoided. But it can be told gently and matter-of-factly, without the use of the professional's own reactive adjectives. "I know this will be a shock to you, but your child has a condition called spina bifida. She has problems with nerve damage to the lower legs, bladder and bowel, and she also has a build-up of fluid in her head called hydrocephalus." How different this sounds from, "This child will always be a hopeless cripple: she will never walk or run or have bowel and bladder control, and she may be retarded as well." It should not take much stretching of the imagination to realize the differences in effect that these kinds of statements can have. Naturally, each aspect of the situation needs to be explained more fully in terms the parent can understand. But to convey by word or attitude that the child is worthless, hopeless, or grotesque is to allow one's own difficulties in dealing with the problem to poison the situation in a most unprofessional manner.

But what, exactly, *is* "the truth"? Immediately, all the problems of predicting future outcomes for an individual child come into play. Certainly, the parents need to have outlined for them the general dimensions of the problem. This is best done all at once. The parent who is told in "dribs and drabs" over days or weeks may continue to be plagued by the fear of "what is he or she holding back from me this time?" Such a fear interferes with the ability to trust what the professional is saying. The facts, difficult as they may be, can nevertheless be easier to cope with than the uncertainty as to whether something even worse is looming just over the horizon.

This does not necessarily mean presenting every possible implication of every problem in the initial session. I can recall very clearly listening to an earnest young resident discussing my daughter's

condition of spina bifida when she was just a few days old, until he
began to talk at length about the social implications of incontinence
in the school-age child. I suddenly found myself standing next to the
isolette nodding my head intelligently (or so I hoped) and not hearing
another word that he said. Although I knew that the nerves to her
bladder had been affected, I simply had not, and could not, think
through to the details of what that would mean in future years.

In many cases, it will be difficult, if not impossible, to predict
how the child will fare in the future. The best that can be done is to
be prepared with the most recent medical and treatment information,
and to admit honestly that which is not known.

The whole truth must include not only the problems of the child
but also what is positive in the situation. For the newborn, it may be
simply something like "she has a strong, healthy cry" or "she seems to
be alert and responsive to being held and cuddled." For an older child,
it may be whatever she does well or shows more strengths in. Often,
the picture that fills the parent's mind is far bleaker than the reality.
Some parents of children who are retarded have reported wishing they
had been told that the child would smile, or communicate simple
wishes like wanting a drink of water when thirsty. Other positive
aspects of the situation include what treatments are possible for the
child and what supports (such as parent groups) are available for the
parents.

Parents need to be able to have a sense of what constructive
action can be taken. This can be a powerful help in not becoming
engulfed in feelings of hopelessness and helplessness. To hear "What
this baby needs right *now* is . . . " provides an anchor on which to
begin to cope in a positive way. This can be as simple and as basic as
"What this baby needs now is to be held and fed and loved," if no
immediate surgical or medical treatments are needed.

Lastly, the parent needs and deserves some expression of
compassion; some recognition on the part of the professional person
that this is indeed a severe blow and that he or she will undoubtedly
experience painful reactions to it. One can reach out, as one human
being to another, and acknowledge the pain. This does not mean
attempting to be a psychotherapist to the new parent. It may simply
mean a touch on the shoulder, a phrase of recognition, or the provision
of some private time and space for the parents to be alone, away from
the hustle and bustle of the hospital ward or busy clinic.

The flood of emotions and feelings that engulfs parents as they
first learn of a child's disability makes it impossible for them to attend
fully to the information they may be receiving. The parents simply
cannot hear and incorporate too many things at once. It is necessary
to provide opportunities for repetition and ample time for the parents

to evolve their questions and bring them back for answers. Written explanations and instructions which the parents can take home and refer to as they need to or are able to are useful.

And questions there will be, as the parents struggle to understand what has happened, why it has happened, what they need to do about it, and what it will mean both to the child and to their own lives. Up-to-date and factual information presented in the context of the evolution of knowledge and understanding of disabilities and birth defects is essential. Glib and blanket statements ("This is one chance in a million" or "Go ahead and have another child — this can't happen to you again") have no place here.

The professional person should have no fears about acknowledging what he or she does not know, and suggesting other referrals or resources for information. Such honesty and willingness to help locate necessary information will win far more respect and trust than will a facade of certainty erected to mask a lack of knowledge.

It is important to stress, whether asked directly or not, what is known about cause in a positive light. A statement such as "Current research has not indicated that anything you did or did not do during this pregnancy caused this condition" can help to ease parental feelings of guilt and responsibility.

The manner in which the professional person relates to the child can have an important impact on the parent. By talking about and reacting to the child as a person rather than as a "defect" or a "condition" one can model and demonstrate acceptance of the child as a child. This only works, however, if it is genuine. Phoniness and pretense will only increase the gap between the parent and the professional and decrease the likelihood that they will be able to work together for the benefit of the child.

The moment of diagnosis may have a somewhat different meaning for the parent who has long suspected that her child has a problem. This parent has been on a cruel roller coaster of alternating hope and despair. She has seized upon each bit of progress of the child, each reassurance of friends, relatives, and professionals that the lags she has noticed may represent normal variations in development, as a basis upon which to pin his hopes that all is, after all, well; only to experience again and again the recurrence of her own anxiety and growing conviction that this is not so.

The pain of having her hopes irrevocably crushed is indeed great, and her sorrow for the child is acute. But at the same time, there may be some small element of relief in learning the nature of the problem. Now he no longer needs to flail about ineffectually at ghosts of possible problems (and perhaps be thought by friends and relatives to be over-dramatizing, or making mountains out of molehills). There is now something real to be dealt with, and it becomes possible to make plans and to take actions to deal with the situation.

What *are* the pieces of this thing we call acceptance? What, exactly, are we talking about when we use the term? Acceptance of the child? Or of the fact of the disability? Do we mean resignation, passivity, or a dogged determination to "make the best of it"?

First there is the question of acknowledging that it has happened. The disability is real, and it is present in my child. This may occur in as short a time as moments, as the initial denial — "It can't be, not my child" — has passed. The situation rapidly becomes more complex, however. The condition itself may be acknowledged and admitted, but what exactly one is being asked to accept may remain very unclear. Often, little can be said with great certainty in early infancy. Yes, we may know that a baby is retarded, but do we really know what that will mean in terms of what he will be able to do or learn as an adult? In the case of a condition like spina bifida, we may know that a certain degree of paralysis exists. But at this point the parent is likely to hear a great many qualifying phrases: "*If* hydrocephalus develops," "*If* we can avoid shunt complications," "*If* the hips do not become dislocated," "*If* the kidneys can be kept healthy," and so on. The parent may feel as though he were swimming in a sea of "ifs," and want desperately to find something concrete to hold on to.

For some parents, of course, the stage of denial may last considerably longer. Denial is more difficult (although certainly not impossible) to maintain when the problem is a visible physical one. It may be that these parents will need time to absorb the information, and to observe for themselves the evidence that the child has a problem. Prolonged denial exists because it meets a strong need in the parent not to face the reality of the disability, and may require professional help.

The literature by parents and those who have worked with many parents is replete with instances of parents who have received unduly pessimistic pronouncements of their child's potential. Many of these parents refused to "accept" these gloomy prognoses and continued to battle for something better for their children. And, in retrospect, many of them were right.

One of the most difficult issues for parents to resolve is the question of knowing what must be accepted and what must be challenged and fought for the child's benefit. There *is* a time not to accept too readily or too early definitive statements on prognosis or treatment potentials. There *is* a time to search and to fight for something better. Knowledge of causation and treatment of various conditions is increasing all the time, and there are serious time lags in the dissemination of new information to practicing professionals throughout the country.

Many parents will not be able to "accept" until they have tried everything that they can think of to try. Some will become like the newspaper reporter who lives with the conviction that the hottest story of his career is only on the next block. If only he can move a little faster, search a little harder, perhaps he won't miss it. Thus these parents will continue to devour the literature, and travel to yet another clinic, yet another doctor, and try yet another training program. It can be difficult to say just when this searching is no longer realistic.

Our society's openness and attitudes toward people with disabilities is changing. Gradually, opportunities are increasing, and people with disabilities are being recognized as people with rights and abilities instead of people who need pity and charity. Who has instigated and fought for these changes? For the most part, it has been the disabled themselves and their parents who have refused to accept the status quo and have pressured, lobbied, and fought for social change.

The question of acceptance cannot be looked at in a vacuum. It must be evaluted in terms of the knowledge as it exists at the moment, remembering how much is yet unknown to us; in terms of the interactions of the people involved; and in terms of the social context in which the situation occurs.

There are, nonetheless, natural, normal, and predictable human reactions that occur in parents as they struggle to incorporate the disability of a child into their lives. While these are expected and necessary responses, they also harbor the potential for difficulty if the parent is not able to "work through" to some degree of resolution of each of them.

Once the initial disbelief of shocked denial has passed, the parent experiences an overwhelming grief. Many writers have likened this to the grief experienced with the death of a loved one and have described this in terms of the death of the longed-for "perfect" child who has not been born.

All of us invest in our unborn children many of our own deepest needs and wishes. The anticipated child represents an extension of ourselves, but with fresh potentials, unlimited horizons, and new opportunities. She, we are sure, will have what we felt we did not. Children may represent to the world that we are indeed complete, adult, and mature human beings. We offer our "perfect" children as proof of this fact. The parent of the healthy newborn can gaze at her offspring and retain this vision of the wonder of great talents and unlimited dreams.

This is not so for the parent whose child is born with a disability. The dream is abruptly shattered. Her own competence as a mature adult capable of producing children is suddenly threatened. Parents who are young and healthy, and who are in the midst of a hopeful building of careers, family, and home may suffer also the sudden loss of youth and innocence.

But the grief is not just for the lost dreams. As the parent looks down upon the real child who begins life with a handicap, he grieves at least as much for the present child as for the one who did not appear. The parent can foresee all the pain and the deprivation that he imagines this child will experience. Her tears flow for this child, and what this child has lost. At this time, it may be next to impossible for the parent to conceive of this child experiencing joy, of her going to school, laughing, and playing, and blowing out birthday candles. She thinks only of what cannot be, the legs that will not dance, or the mind that will not study science.

At this stage, the best person to introduce the notion that joys are indeed possible for both the child and her parents is another parent. Professional attempts to do this, while necessary, are more apt to be dismissed because "you don't really know what it feels like." The new parent cannot so readily dismiss the words of another parent, who has lived through the same experience and who can gently assure the new parent that both growth and happiness are indeed possible.

While it is certainly useful for the parent and for the professional working with the parent to recognize and allow for the natural progression of grief and mourning, the process of acceptance for an individual parent and family involves more than this. The emphasis on the mourning reaction, says Ross,

> tends to neglect the fact that the recognition of a discrepancy between the anticipated child and the reality of the defective child represents a crisis and that each person has his own mode of coping with crises. This mode is a response learned in earlier crisis situations and thus depends not only on the individual's personality but also on the implicit meaning the defective child's birth has to the parent.[5]

Thus the grief has different meanings and expressions for different people. The outward behavior of the parent, which may range from a grim stoicism to uncontrolled sobbing, will depend in part on those meanings and in part on the parent's personality and previous experiences with crises.

Time and the experience of growing to know and love the child will help to ease the passage of the acute phase of grief. A residual of sorrow, called "chronic sorrow" by Olshansky,[6] remains, however. Chronic sorrow may lie dormant and unnoticed for long periods of time only to surge forth unexpectedly. It may be simply looking out one's window to see a little girl skipping home from school on a crisp fall day, blithely kicking piles of red and yellow leaves, which brings the almost forgotten tears to a parent's eyes months or years after all the tears were thought to have been shed.

Chronic sorrow, however, may in the long run be more easily incorporated into a parent's life than chronic anxiety. Some disabling conditions have a high potential for unexpected crises. In spina bifida with hydrocephalus, for example, the possibility of malfunction of a shunt (the tube that carries spinal fluid from the ventricles or spaces of the brain to another part of the body where it may safely be reabsorbed) is constant, and when it occurs, it often requires immediate surgery with all the usual risks and possible complications. To make matters worse, each ordinary cold or flu that the child catches may produce headaches similar to those caused by shunt problems. Somehow, the family must find a way to deal realistically with the crises when they do occur and to live the rest of their lives without constant fear. This is not an easy task.

Anxiety about paying high costs for the child's care and treatment, or about what will become of the child who will not be able to be fully independent as an adult when her parents can no longer provide assistance, may be a constant theme in the life of a family. These anxieties arise not from the parent's own internal reactions but from the failure of our society to provide adequately for the needs of its members with disabilities. Anxiety, as a chronic stress for parents, has a high potential for leading to later difficulties.

The issue of parental guilt feelings, however unjustified by objective "facts," is an important one. Perhaps if we humans did not take such inordinate pride in producing healthy, beautiful offspring, we would not be so devastated by guilt feelings when something goes wrong.

Many parents experience a compelling need to search for the causes and explanations of the child's problem. Some of this stems from a need to look for possible evidence of wrongdoing of some kind. The events of the pregnancy may be reviewed over and over in the search for clues. Whether or not the prospective parents were happy to learn of the pregnancy, elements of the mother's diet, any possible evidence of illness, or any activities in which the mother feels she perhaps should not have participated all come under scrutiny.

Factual information about what is known about the causes of the child's problem will do much to alleviate unnecessary and possibly debilitating guilt. But some may remain, for not all of the guilt is entirely rational or logical. The mother who carried the child for 9 long months, who felt it begin to move and kick, and whose body nourished and nurtured the child, may feel a deep and lasting sense of responsibility even when she "knows" intellectually that there was nothing that she could have done to alter the outcome.

The issue of who or what is to blame for the condition may be agonizing for all concerned, particularly if the disability is thought to be an accident or injury of birth. The question "Why did this happen?" is a compelling one, and the search for its resolution may lead families into a mutually suspicious search into each parent's family tree, or into blaming the persons present at the birth. Unanswerable questions are difficult to live with. Acknowledging these feelings, and openly but gently discussing what is known about the situation can help to minimize unjustified and possibly harmful blame-seeking.

Parents in their anguish may direct their questions and their anger at fate, at the universe, or at God. To think, "If God is good he would not have done this to this innocent child" may be, for the parent who considers herself to be a religious person, an unacceptable thought. As Ross puts it, "This question is unacceptable to a religious person and the doubt of divine wisdom it implies creates guilt."[5] The very premises on which she has built her life may be shaken by such doubts.

Anger is a perfectly normal and natural response when a child becomes disabled. When nature or fate has, capriciously it seems, selected this particular child to begin life with a disability, a deep rage at the unfairness of it wells up in the parent. Parents may also be angry at the effects on their own lives: the awesome responsibility that looms ahead, the necessity to change their life plans, and the destruction of their dreams. But where should they direct this anger? At fate? At God? At the doctors? Often, none of the choices seems quite appropriate. Like the unanswerable questions, the parent is left with a seemingly unresolvable but powerful feeling.

These feelings and reactions are especially acute in the first weeks and months of their child's disability. Time and understanding will help in their resolution, but the feelings are powerful. They may slip below the surface to appear, perhaps in altered form, later on.

Anger may be channeled into vigorous efforts on the child's behalf. It may lead parents into advocacy and voluntary group efforts to be an effective force in working for better treatment and opportunities for people with disabilities. But anger can also work slowly, below the surface, to present problems in the lives of parents. Parents may feel very guilty about admitting, even to themselves, that they feel anger about the effects of the disability and its demands on their own lives. Somehow, it seems unworthy to acknowledge that one feels that way: "After all, the disability happened to my child, not to me. She is the one who really has to put up with the problems," the parent will say. It is important for parents to know that these feelings are normal and natural, and that the door is open for discussion of them.

It may be useful, in discussing issues of acceptance, to be clear whether we are discussing acceptance of the *child* or the *disability*. It is essential for the child's growth and development that she be accepted into the family. It may be relatively easy in the case of a physical disability conceptually to separate the child as a person from the disability that has happened to her. In the case of the child who is retarded, this becomes more difficult because our ideas and feelings about "people" are so intricately involved with aspects of intelligence and personality.

For some parents, initial acceptance of the child as a member of the family is not an issue at all. To them, as they stand looking at their newborn child, belongs the certainty that "She is ours. We will do the best we can to love her, care for her, and raise her." Their children are, without hesitation, incorporated immediately into the matrix of the family.

This certainty may be based on religious faith or personal philosophy. The depth of the parents' sorrow may be no less; their acceptance may be sorely tested as the realities of the child's limitations unfold with time; but there is no question that she is one of them.

But even parents of perfectly "normal" infants do not always immediately or automatically respond with great rushes of maternal or paternal love. It may take time to adjust to the reality of a new human being, and of being a parent. Certainly, our "traditional" birth procedures, with the mother sedated, the father in a waiting room down the hall, and the baby whisked away to the nursery, have served in the past to discourage these very early attachments to the new member of the family.

The work done by Klaus and Kennell[7] on maternal-infant bonding indicates that there may be a sensitive period immediately after birth for such attachments to occur. They report that movements of the mother and child in the first few minutes and hours of life are mutual and synchronized. It is known that if this sensitive period is missed in certain species of animals, mother-child bonding will not take place. Certainly, humans do have the capacity to compensate for this lack, but we may make it harder for ourselves by not providing for this whenever possible. It may be extremely difficult for the family whose child is immediately removed to an intensive care unit or even to another more specialized hospital to form the necessary attachments.

It is also difficult for some people, according to Klaus and Kennel, to experience attachment and mourning at the same time. The mother who is grieving for the loss of a loved one (her own parent, perhaps) at the time of birth may experience more difficulty in becoming attached to her child. The grieving experienced by the parent of the child with a disability may also interfere with the bonding process.

The parent may undergo "anticipatory grief" for the death of the infant if this is a possibility.

My own daughter was born just a few days before Christmas, and remained in the hospital when I returned home 2 days later. I had held her for only a few moments when she was 8 hours old, just prior to her first surgery. At home on Christmas Day, immediately after the obligatory but joyless turkey dinner, my husband brought me my coat. When I asked where he wanted to go, he said "To the hospital." Resisting, I replied, "But it won't make any difference to her. She is only 4 days old." My pain was too acute and too much my own to allow any reaching out to my child. I felt that if I became attached to her and *then* she died, it would be unbearable.

My husband insisted, and eventually prevailed. We arrived in the intensive care nursery to discover that her isolette was decorated with tiny stockings and Christmas ornaments. The nurses talked to her by name, cooing and commenting proudly on her eating as they placed her in my lap. No one lectured to me, but their actions pierced my pain with the awareness that this infant was indeed a very real person, and my daughter. The skies did not part, and no bolt of lightning appeared, but my commitment to her and my love for her had taken root.

The process of acceptance is a long one. Each new phase of the child's development will pose new aspects and new challenges. Each new piece of evidence of society's acceptance or lack of acceptance of the disability presents yet another need for reaction of some sort. Parents may be surprised to find, as their disabled teenager weeps about being excluded by the admired "in" group, that feelings assumed to be long buried and gone come rising to the surface with just as much intensity as they had years before.

Acceptance does not mean passive resignation. It means continuing to struggle and to challenge to find the best possible for the child and the family. Realistic acceptance acknowledges that "negative" feelings of anger and sadness are natural and will continue to be felt, although they will assume different proportions as enthusiasm, hope, and joy resume their places in the parents' lives. It may even lead one into battle with what is unacceptable in our society. The professional person will find that the parent with this kind of acceptance may be far from docile.

QUESTIONS FOR PARENTS

These are questions designed to assist you — the parents — in sorting out your thoughts and reactions to your child's problem. They may be difficult questions to think about. Do not expect to answer them fully or immediately. As you think about your answers, you may be shocked or disappointed by some of your "gut" responses. Do not ignore these or be ashamed of them; be assured that these only illustrate your "humanness" and that other parents who have dealt successfully with this situation have had these feelings too. You can expect your thoughts and feelings to shift over time. As you have the courage to face your honest reactions, you may be able to see ways that you can incorporate this knowledge into yourself and to grow from having done so. Looking at feelings, not burying them, is the way to become free from burdens of guilt or anger. You may also be able to recognize when you could benefit from sharing these feelings with your spouse, a trusted friend, another parent, or a professional counselor or therapist.

1. What were my dreams and fantasies for this child?
2. What did I hope this child would mean to me in my own life?
3. What do I think my child has lost because of this disability or problem?
4. What do I think *I* have lost because of this disability?
5. Can I look at my child and see him or her as a person, not as a diagnosis?
6. How do I feel about accepting the demands that I see being placed on me?
7. How can I deal with the unanswerable questions, the uncertainties of the future?
8. Do I see any possibility that the experience of raising this child can enrich my life? My family's?
9. Do I know where I can look for help, for the child, and for myself?

REFERENCES

1. Barsch, Ray H., *The Parent of the Handicapped Child*, Charles C. Thomas, 1969.
2. Meadows, Kathryn, Parental Responses to Medical Ambiguities of Deafness, *Journal of Health and Social Behavior*, December, 1968.
3. Roos, P., A Parent's View of What Public Education Should Accomplish, in *Educational Programming for the Severely and Profoundly Handicapped*, E. Sontag, Ed., Council for Exceptional Children, 1977.
4. Brown, S. L. and Moersch, M., Eds., *Parents on the Team*, University of Michigan Press, 1978.
5. Ross, Alan O., *The Exceptional Child in the Family*, Grune and Stratton, 1964.
6. Olshansky, Simon, Chronic Sorrow: A Response to Having a Mentally Defective Child, *Social Casework*, April 1962.
7. Klaus, Marshall H. and Kennell, John H., *Maternal-Infant Bonding*, C. V. Mosby, 1976.

2
IMPACT ON THE FAMILY SYSTEM

The child with a disability is not just born to a parent, or even to two parents. He or she is an addition to an ongoing, interlocking family unit. Although each child has two biological parents, these family units come in many shapes and forms. We cannot afford to think solely in terms of mother, father, and two children. Divorced parents, blended families, and single-parent families are increasingly common in today's world. Regardless of the size and composition of a particular family unit, each will define itself as a "family." A family may already include other children when a child with a disability is born. Grandparents, other relatives, or close friends may be included in the family unit or they may be more peripheral to it.

The story of the family's life does not begin with the birth of a child with a disability. Each family has a history. Each has its own established patterns of interaction and operation. Understanding the impact that a child's disability has on a family requires that one have some sense of how families grow and function.

The literature of the family therapy field reveals that family therapists have found it helpful to think of family organization and functioning in systems terms. Families operate as systems in a number of ways. Using the language of these systems characteristics makes it possible to think and talk about families with all of their richness and individual variation. Some of the ways in which families can be said to function as systems follow.

"WHOLENESS" AND BOUNDARIES

The "whole" of a family is greater than the sum of its parts. Families are more than collections of individuals. They have an atmosphere, a character, which is somehow greater than and different from the characteristics and personalities of their members. Although difficult to define, this "essence" of the family may be sensed and felt. The family has a flavor, almost a personality, that is uniquely its own and different from other families.

One of the ways in which this sense of "wholeness" is maintained is through the definition of who is in the family and who is not. Each family has boundaries in some shape or form. Some people are defined as belonging to the family unit, and others are not. In some families, boundaries are tight and clear-cut. These families may be very self-sufficient and self-contained. In other families, boundaries are looser and more easily permeated. People tend to move more easily in and out of these families. Such a family may from time to time include grandparents, relatives, or close friends who may live with the family for a period of time. Or they may take in foster children or others in need of a home.

INTERRELATIONSHIP OF PARTS

Members of a family unit are interlocking parts of the system. Each part of the system is connected to each other part by a continuous feedback loop. Behavior of a person in the family is not only a stimulus *for* another person but is also at the same time a response *to* that other person. No comment or action comes "out of the blue;" each has a relationship to what has gone before. The patterns of relationships are continuous and mutual. To attempt to say that one person's actions "cause" a response in another is to miss half of the pattern, because the action is itself already a response. If a wife says she nags her husband because he drinks, and he says he drinks because she nags, can either be right?

The communication connections between people in the family are both verbal and nonverbal. Tone of voice, body posture, and facial expression are all important ways we communicate nonverbally. Powerful messages can be transmitted without words. We know, for example, that children can be exquisitely sensitive to underlying messages such as, "You are a worthwhile person, and though I must punish this behavior I know you are capable of learning and growing," or "Basically, you are a bad person and I must punish you to prevent you from acting as bad as you really are."

These connections, both spoken and unspoken, between family members are important in understanding what goes on in a family. Each member is affected by the experience of another; and each has an impact on the others as well. Events and reactions do not happen just to one individual; ripples of effect are felt throughout the system.

RULES AND BALANCE

Each family has evolved over time a series of rules which govern how the people will operate in that family. Certain behaviors are allowed in the family, while others are not. Some rules may be very explicit (such as who handles what chores in the family, or how much children are allowed to "talk back" to the parents). Other rules are more implicit. Powerful rules against talking about certain subjects may be operating in a family without anyone ever having said aloud that this was not to be discussed. Somehow, everyone in the family "knows" that sex or Mother's nervous breakdown are not to be talked about.

There may also be rules about rules, or, rules for ways in which the family can change the rules. One of the ways in which families can get stuck in unsatisfactory or painful patterns of interactions is that they do not have ways to change the rules or to renegotiate how they will deal with each other. Family members may notice, for example, that Father has become increasingly tense and short-tempered. But if the rules are that Father's moods are not to be talked about, the family will have no way openly to react to and deal with this situation. Families may continue to operate under old rules when new ones might be more appropriate, when children have grown to new stages of development, for example.

Families seek to maintain a homeostasis, or a balance, in their operations and functioning. If one person becomes ill, others will take over his or her tasks. If a behavior (such as a fight between the parents) threatens to escalate out of control, the family will have ways to halt that escalation and return things to their normal state. Mother may cry, or Father may walk out to "cool off" for a few hours. Some families set their internal thermostats on "high," letting their emotions and feelings flow freely; while others operate on a much "cooler" setting.

Because of the interlocking nature of the family as a system, a stress experienced anywhere in that system will have effects everywhere as the system reacts and shifts to restore itself to a balanced state. The point at which a stress "shows up" as a problem may not be where the trouble is at all. It is well-known in the family therapy field, for example, that a child who is brought to a counselor because he has a behavior problem may be a clue to the fact that there is a hidden battle going on between the parents.

The birth of a child with a disability can represent a severe stress to the family system. Each parent reacts not only to the event and to what it means to him or her as an individual, but also to the reactions of other persons who are important in the system. Often, parents' reactions may seem to be opposite: when one feels despair, the other sees hope.

Or, when one withdraws, the other more fully throws himself or herself into the child's activities or therapy programs. Each may feel that the other does not fully understand or fully accept what the child's situation is. Each may feel lonely and misunderstood. For some, this may be their first experience with the essential loneliness of human grief and pain.

The view of the family as a continuing, interrelated system provides a somewhat different perspective. The family as a functioning entity attempts to maintain its stability in the face of stress and crisis. If all the members of the family were to succumb to despair at the same time, family functioning might cease. Families that become caught in painful patterns may benefit from exploring different ways of restoring their equilibrium. The father who "buries" himself in work to pay the bills for his disabled child may seem to be impatient with his depressed wife who is preoccupied with worries and fears for the child. Underneath, he may fully share those worries and fears but be afraid that if he "gives in" to his own depression like his wife, the family will fall apart. A new balance of sharing might allow the father to express more feeling and become more involved with his child, and free the mother from her role as "sole mourner" so that she can utilize her energies to contribute more to the family.

SYSTEMS WITHIN SYSTEMS

Even as the family as a whole can be considered as a system, other groupings of people within the family can be identified. These are known as subsystems. For example, the parents as a couple are one such subsystem. Parents are spouses, partners, and lovers to each other as well as parents to their children. The quality of this relationship is a crucial one; in most families, it sets the tone and style for the rest of the family. It may be helpful both for those who live in families and those who wish to understand families and the impact of stress to focus separately on the different relationships within the family. A common pitfall for parents who are besieged by worries and demands is that of neglecting to nurture their relationship to each other.

The children, as a group, constitute another subsystem. When one of the children is disabled and requires special help or frightening medical treatments, the relationship between brothers and sisters is affected. Other groupings can be identified: mother-daughters, father-sons, and so forth.

The family, of course, also has a place in larger systems. These are made up of the extended family (grandparents, aunts, uncles and cousins), the neighborhood and community, and the larger society. Here too, many patterns are possible. The family may be quite self-contained and independent, or it may have close ties to relatives, neighborhood, and external social systems. The needs of a handicapped child may make it necessary for a family to change its relationship to the outside world. Suddenly, the family cannot meet all the needs of this child as it does for its other children. It must look to others for various kinds of treatment and assistance. Help may be needed to pay the bills. It may even be necessary to ask others to come into the home to help care for other children while the parents take the child who has the disability to the hospital.

Thus the birth, or the diagnosis, of a child with a disability has a profound impact on all levels of the family system. Because the system is interconnected, events and reactions in one part of the system have effects of some sort on all parts. Each person in that system reacts not only to what has happened, but also to how others in the family are reacting. The family may grow and be strengthened as it learns to cope with the situation, or it may founder if its coping mechanisms cannot successfully meet the demands. Many families do both.

It may be difficult for some families to incorporate the severely disabled child within its boundaries. The usual bonding process between parent and child may have been interfered with because of physical separation of the child in the hospital. The family may have strong unspoken values such as "We are strong. We are healthy; we are of good sturdy stock." In previous years, families were even encouraged to reject children who were defective. When I was a student nurse, the newborn nursery usually contained at least one infant with Down's syndrome who was left behind by the family, sight unseen, to await placement in an institution.

Each individual in the family system will experience his or her own reactions to this event. Each parent brings to the experience his or her own personality, self-image, and dreams. Some of our ideals, fantasies, and dreams are not clear to our conscious minds, so that aspects of our feelings and our grief are mysterious and perhaps even firghtening in their intensity. The demands of raising this child look like none we have ever been called upon to meet before. "Oh, no," we think, "I cannot possibly do that." Our previous experiences do not look as though they will be of much help to us.

Other children in the family will observe their parents' grief. They will feel the tension and worry, and they may puzzle over what it means. If mother is suddenly spending long hours in the hospital with the baby, they may feel lonely and unloved. As they begin to understand the problems that their brother or sister has, they will experience their own grief, worry, and guilt. They will probably feel guilty about their own feelings of resentment. Parents may suddenly seem to expect them to become more independent, more "grown up."

They may have to help with household chores and not bother Mommy with as many requests. The fortunate ones will be able to share in the grief of their parents and be able to give as well as receive comfort.

The family may well have rules about how to act in a crisis. These may be unspoken, but understood by all as "this is the way we handle things." For many families, the stiff upper lip is expected to be maintained at all times, especially in contacts with people outside the household. If families have strong rules about not feeling sorry for oneself, it may be difficult for family members to allow themselves to recognize and deal with the impact of the disability on their own lives. Some things are just not talked about in some families. Fears about the child's death or about the parent's own sense of inadequacy may have to be ignored or buried if the parent is to keep from breaking the family rules.

All of the relationships in the subsystems of the family are affected in one way or another. These effects are not necessarily negative. The older child who is required to take a more active part in the running of the household and teaming up with Mom and Dad, for example, may discover a whole new sense of self-esteem through his expanded roles as helper and competent assistant. Change, however, *will* occur. A sense of the family as an interconnected whole can help us to have a better awareness of changes that are healthy and positive and those that are not.

The relationship between the parents alters with the birth of any child, particularly the first. The stress of the disability of a child adds additional dimensions which may prove difficult. Each spouse may have looked to the other for the supports and strengths that he or she needed to cope with the world. Suddenly, each may be faced with needs so great that he or she cannot possibly meet the needs of the other. Each may need the other to be strong and to provide comfort and stability. Each may be working so hard to "control" his own internal fears and anxieties that he cannot bear to hear the other voice these questions.

While it is entirely true that a crisis may be beneficial in the sense that it may galvanize a family's strengths and bring the members together in a common battle, prolonged stress is a very different matter. Repeated crises tend to erode and wear down coping ability and to increase the separation between marital partners as each tries desperately to hold onto his own strengths.

Even the sexual relationshp between the parents may be affected in a variety of ways. Sex can be a vivid reminder: "This is how it happened." If there are any hidden traces of guilt over present or past sexual activities, these may be activated by the fact of the disability.

Old ideas about punishment for sins can persist long after we think
we know that they are not rational or logical.

Satisfying sexual relationships require a basic sense of self-worth,
"I am an attractive and worthwhile person." This sense of self-esteem
can be badly shaken by the fact of having produced a defective child.
Feelings of inability to cope with the situation weaken the sense of
mastery and competence.

Guilt feelings that may be rationally and logically discounted in
other areas of life may crop up when it is time for sex. "How can I
enjoy myself and 'have fun' in the midst of this tragedy?"

Parents, of course, may also be simply too drained, too fatigued
by the stress and the demands of caring for the child to have the energy
to comfort and to give pleasure to each other. There may be little
respite for the demands; if the child is ill or does not sleep well at night,
the parent may be "on duty" 24 hours a day.

Anger brewing between the parents may show up first in the
sexual relationship. The mother may feel that her husband does not
really understand the child's problem or that he has "deserted" her,
leaving her to do all the caretaking and worrying for the child. Or the
father may feel that his wife is overemotional, overanxious, and too
involved with the child. Underneath, he may feel very needful of
nurturing himself.

We know that families do not remain static over time. In fact,
the demands on a family to change and adapt in the natural course
of events are strong and inevitable. Young couples face the tasks of
establishing a new household, achieving independence from their own
families, and providing for their own security and development. As
children are added to the family, the couple must learn to be parents
as well as spouses. Children grow and change rapidly, and each new
stage of development calls for changes and shifts in the family balance.
Finally, the family, having prepared the children as best it can to make
their way in the world, must send them on their way to establish their
own separate lives and families.

Families are expected, in our culture, to provide for the basic
practical needs of living. The provision of food, shelter, clothing, and
the management of the outside world constitutes a major part of the
activities within a given household. Meals must be prepared, taxes
and bills must be paid, and children must have clean clothing and
lunch money as they leave for school each day. Families are also
expected to provide the emotional support, restoration, and nurturing
that will enable their members to cope and hold their own in the
world. Needs for intimacy and for the sexual satisfaction of parents
are, for the most part, expected to be met within the family.

Within these overall goals and expectations, the individual family's priorities and needs will shift as it progresses through the usual developmental stages of life. We are used to thinking of developmental stages of childhood; we are less accustomed to thinking about such stages in the lives of adults and of families. Such a perspective is useful in understanding the impact of a child's disability on the parents and on the family as a whole. We are not the same throughout our adult lives; our needs and our perspectives change as we progress from our twenties into our thirties, forties, fifties, and beyond.

Young parents are involved in establishing themselves as independent, capable adults. They may still be working out a new relationship with their own parents in which they will shift from being children to being adults. The birth of a child with a disability may mean that they suddenly must turn again to their own parents for assistance, whether it be for emotional support, financial help, or child care. Their newly found ability to manage their own lives seems suddenly in jeopardy, and it may be difficult to accept needed help from the child's grandparents.

Young parents are also usually very involved in establishing themselves in the career and work world. Their concepts of themselves as competent and capable people may be shaken. At home, they are faced with heavy demands, crises, and the worry that they may not be able to do or to be all that will be required of them. It is difficult to leave at home feelings of being unable to cope with a sick, hyperactive or needful child when they go to a job or office.

Young adulthood is a time of continuing to build a self-concept. This sense of oneself as reasonably attractive and competent may be threatened. As one mother said to me, "Somehow, having one's handicapped child lumbering and clomping slowly behind oneself detracts from one's own image of oneself. [For me], it takes away from my feelings of being attractive, or a relatively free person. In a sense, I feel restricted, trapped, pulled on, and ugly." These are not pretty feelings, and it takes a great deal of courage to be able to acknowledge having them.

This mother goes on to say, "To confront those feelings makes one feel like a 'bad person,' a 'bad and unacceptable mother'. And, if you don't like yourself, you are not much good to anyone." For this mother, and for many of us who are parents, the recognition of such "awful" feelings led to feeling even worse: because we had to admit that we were the kind of people who could feel that way. Emerging from this potentially self-destructive pattern requires an acceptance of oneself as a truly human person, subject to the same weaknesses and frailties of all humans. These kinds of feelings and reactions are normal and natural; if they can be looked at and shared —

with a spouse, other parents, or a professional counselor — they can lose their power to sap self-esteem further.

Young parents who are expecting children must make plans for the care of those children. The parents may have adopted a traditional "split" of duties, in which the father earns the income in the years that the children are young while the mother stays home to do the bulk of the child care. Or, today's parents may have agreed upon different combinations of mother and father sharing both wage-earning and child care. The woman who has decided to continue her own career may have developed elaborate plans for child care and ways to balance the demands of both work and home. Suddenly, all the carefully detailed plans may not work. The usual child care arrangements of day-care or babysitters may not be possible when there is need for frequent trips to doctors and clinics, exercises, special care, and emergencies beyond the usual childhood infections and accidents.

Difficult decisions must be made as the young family tries to adapt to these demands. The question may become one of which parent's career comes first, or who can obtain a job with flexible enough hours to allow for the extra care and emergencies. Plans and agreements which were laboriously and painstakingly worked out must often be scrapped.

If the child with a disability is the first-born, the tasks may be even more difficult. These parents do not "know" that they are capable of producing healthy offspring because they have not done so. They may be less able than the parent who already has one or two "normal" children to accept the disability as an accident of nature rather than a profound statement of their own inadequacies. The questions relating to having further children can be agonizing, and require factual and up-to-date information and genetic counseling provided in a sensitive manner.

One of the tasks of the early stages of family development is that of the new parents learning how to be parents, to care for and to teach their children. The parents who already have other children have some experience "under their belts." They have some knowledge of the usual stages of child development and a sense of their own ability to manage successfully. The parents whose child with a disability is the first-born do not have this experience to guide them. When the newborn requires specialized medical and nursing care, the new parents may feel even more helpless and inept. The mother who is not permitted to hold and care for her infant because of his health needs and who can only stand and look at him in the isolette may feel that she is even dangerous to the child.[1] It is important in such situations that the parents be given support and encouragement to care for their children in the hospital as soon as it is medically feasible.

Families in the middle stages of development have usually passed beyond the initial stages of establishing the family and providing for its basic needs. Now, questions about the life style of the family are more often addressed. Where they will live, and how they will spend their time and develop their interests become concerns. Will they live in an apartment or a house? In the city or in a rural area? Will they be campers, skiers, or musicians? What happens to the family that must choose between a vacation and an appliance or treatment for a child? Or the family of avid skiers that now includes a child in a wheelchair? The choices may be difficult and painful to make.

In the usual progression of family life, the middle years are times when children ordinarily, and often unremarkably, pass various milestones of development. Going off to school for the first time, the first 10-speed bike, and the first paper route or babysitting job are all markers along the road to gradually increasing independence. As the times for each of these events arrives, the parents are reminded of their sorrow and their anger that these things are not to be for this child.

When the child with the disability is the youngest, he is growing up at a time when the parents are already beginning to "launch" their older children into the world. But older children may be needed to help care for their younger brother or sister. They may be held back from their own independence not only by the parents' need for help but also by their own feelings of guilt about being "whole" and having the freedom and ability to do the things that are not possible for their brother or sister.

Parents at this stage of life are ordinarily beginning to look forward to and prepare for the time when their parenting role is over and their children are on their own in the world. Parents may look forward to a smaller house in the country, more travel, or the opportunity to pursue their hobbies in retirement. But parents of a child with a handicap cannot look forward to this freedom. Their child may need assistance throughout his or her life. They will need to remain in the role of parent for the rest of their lives, and will often worry about what will become of the child when they are no longer able to provide the help he needs. Issues of facing one's own aging and approaching death can be difficult in the normal course of events. The sense that one's life work is not completed may make this even more painful.

A number of writers have looked at the developmental stages of family life and have investigated the impact of a disability on those stages. Farber describes the process by which a mentally retarded child affects the family as an arrest in the life cycle.[2] The usual progression halts at the point in childhood where parents are still assuming a good deal of responsibility for the care of the child. Farber also found a greater impact on the marital relationship of the parents when the child was an older retarded boy living at home. If it is reasonable to assume that in the 1950s when this work was done a greater degree of independence was expected of boys than of girls, this tends to support the idea that the widening of the discrepancy between what is usual or desired and what is real is increasingly stressful.

Other work on the effects of retardation on families helps to clarify the critical points at which family stress is likely to be experienced. Wikler outlines these times of exacerbation of parental reactions and stress as the times the child had reached or had passed the usual markers of development. These include the usual ages for walking, talking, starting public school, and the child's twenty-first birthday, which usually signifies the end of childhood and the beginning of more adult independence.[3]

Each of these critical points represents a time when the parent is likely to be very aware that a child is "supposed to" be able to move on to a new stage of development. An infant who is retarded or physically disabled needs much the same care as any other infant; but when he or she is 3 or 4 years old and cannot talk, or walk, or be toilet-trained, the differences are much more visible. The reality of the disability is apparent with a new force at each of these points.

In other work, Wikler and others found that certain structural factors were also related to a family's being at risk for stress. The factors included the birth-order, age, and sex of the child, the social class and religion of the family, and the degree to which the family had supportive family and social networks.[4] Parents who can turn to relatives and friends during times of increased sorrow and pain may be able to cope with these critical points with less difficulty. Birth order of the child seems to be important because in some families, the first-born may symbolize more of the hopes and dreams of the family. The presence of younger children who catch up to, and pass, older retarded siblings in their skills and abilities also highlight the disability.

It seems quite likely that there are also similar critical points in the lives of families with physically handicapped children. Certainly, when the child reaches the age of 2 or 3 and cannot walk or run, this fact is painfully brought home to parents.

Other critical points for families of physically disabled children may be the first school placement, the later latency years, and adolescence. School placement often represents the first real separation of mother and child; and the child's differences may be accentuated by the fact that he is picked up by a special bus instead of walking to the neighborhood school with the other children. As the child child approaches 8 or 10 years of age, his size and weight begin to make it impossible for the parents to lift and carry him as they used to. Now, shopping trips, outings, and vacations must be carefully planned to avoid being "stuck" in inaccessible places. Again, the reality of the disability has a new impact. The years of adolescence for the physically handicapped child, as for children who are mentally retarded, arouse in the parent anxiety about the future and the life it holds for the child, as well as anxiety about the parents' own aging and potential inability to keep helping the child.

All of this may sound grim indeed. The reader may wonder what use it is for parents to know these things. The use is that knowing enables us, to some extent at least, to prepare ourselves psychologically for expected stresses. Some anticipatory preparation *can* help. We can be comforted by knowing that surges of anxiety or sorrow at these times are normal and expected; this knowledge alone reduces some of the anxiety. We can know that we are not helpless, bizarre, or "crazy," but, rather, we are experiencing very natural human reactions.

A very real danger for parents of children with disabilities, however, is that of ignoring signs of trouble in ourselves. We may forget that we are just as likely as anyone else to be subject to various psychological or interpersonal difficulties. Undue anxiety, depression, marital difficulties, alcoholism, or other problems can happen to us as well as our neighbor. And yet, as Heisler points out, families of children with disabilities do not ordinarily seek professional help for their problems.[5] Somehow, we think, our troubles are only natural because of our "problem" — the child — and, of course, we know that that situation cannot be miraculously changed. What we often forget is that while our child may not be able to have the "cure" we would like, we *can* still make changes in how we deal with the stresses and how we help each other within the family.

QUESTIONS FOR PARENTS

1. What are the goals of my family at this stage in our lives?
   a. Short-range: what must we do to survive?
   b. Long-range: what do we want for our future?
2. What does our family value most?
3. What are the "rules" for coping in my family? Would I like to change any of these rules?
4. What are the needs of each individual in the family?
   a. Myself?
   b. My spouse?
   c. Other children?
   d. The child with the disability?
5. Where do the needs conflict?

6. What resources do we have to call upon to meet these needs? (i.e., relatives, professionals, social agencies, our own strengths, parent support groups, etc.)
7. Where are the areas where the resources are not sufficient to meet the needs?
8. What are my options in dealing with these?

REFERENCES

1. Klaus, Marshall H. and Kennell, John H., *Maternal-Infant Bonding*, C.V. Mosby, 1976.
2. Farber, Bernard, Effects of a Severely Mentally Retarded Child on Family Integration, *Monograph of the Society for Research in Child Development*, Vol. 24, No. 2, 1959.
3. Wikler, Lynn, Chronic Stresses, Family Relations, April 1981.
4. Wikler, Lynn; Cox, Jane Banning; Daley, Kathy; Galbraith-Gregory, Jill; Laten, Sherry and Miezio, Peggy, Predicting Stress in Families of Retarded Children, University of Wisconsin — Madison School of Social Work, unpublished.
5. Heisler, Verda, *A Handicapped Child in the Family: A Guide for Parents*, Grune and Stratton, 1972.

3
DEALING WITH OTHER PEOPLE
Family, Friends, and Strangers

The fact of a child's disability permeates every aspect of a parent's life. Nowhere is this more apparent than in the complex web of relationships that parents are already involved in. Parents have relatives, friends, and neighbors; they have employers and colleagues at work; they are continually meeting new people in the course of their daily lives. These contacts with other people can be enriching and supportive or they can be strained and painful.

Parents may wish they could retreat to a desert island to be alone while they come to terms with this new event in their lives. But they cannot; the world does not wait. Grandparents, relatives, and friends want to know what is happening and how they can help, and someone must continue going to work to keep the family afloat financially.

Yet these contacts with other people can be a rich source of support and comfort. How people feel — whether they are depressed, angry, or contented — depends in large part upon the quality of their interactions with others. People who feel misunderstood or cut off from others in their lives are more likely to feel angry or depressed. If, on the other hand, people can be reasonably open and honest in their dealings with others and feel that they are understood, it is less likely that reservoirs of hurt, isolation, or depression will build up to a point which gives them trouble.

Professional people who are concerned with the family's ability to manage its situation successfully would do well to focus not just on the child and the parents as individuals but also on the larger social systems of the extended family and the community in which they live. Families, neighbors, community resources, and other parents of disabled children are rich potential sources of support and learning.

AT BIRTH

Many significant events in our lives represent turning points, or the transition from one phase of life to another. Our society has evolved traditions of rituals and rites for marking these events with celebration or mourning. Births, deaths, graduations, marriages, and retirements all have certain traditional activities associated with them. The rituals of casseroles, condolence calls, cards, and gifts all provide people with mechanisms for reaching out and participating in the joys and sorrows of others.

But there are no rules to follow when a child is born with a handicap. People have no traditional guidelines to look to for advice on how to respond. The usual expressions of congratulations on the occasion of a birth seem inappropriate. The rituals and expressions of death do not fit either. What is left, often, is an awkward silence.

This silence may seem puzzling and hurtful to the parents who are already feeling very isolated by this new experience. Suddenly, the parents feel that they inhabit a different world from that of their relatives and friends. The expected pattern of their lives has been irrevocably altered, and they must adjust to a different set of goals and expectations for this child. The typical concerns of the other young parents who are their friends — worries about feeding, teething, or measles shots — seem trivial and remote to the parents who are visiting their child in an infant intensive care unit.

People who want to reach out but do not know what to say may remain silent for fear of saying the wrong thing. This may become a source of deep hurt for the new parents until they realize, sometimes a long time later, that it can stem not from a lack of caring but rather from a lack of knowledge of what is appropriate or helpful in this kind of situation.

Parents themselves may be unwittingly signaling to their friends, "Don't talk to me about this. I can't discuss it yet." When people's wounds are raw and they are uncertain about their ability to cope, they may attempt to marshall their resources by withdrawing into themselves. To talk about it, they fear, might be to risk total collapse. They may be quite unaware that it is their manner which rebuffs people who might want to reach out to them.

Some people attempt to bridge the gap with comments meant to be an effort to comfort. Often, such efforts seem clumsy and insensitive to parents. Most parents have heard comments like "So-and-so's baby is worse off than yours," "How fortunate he or she is to have been born to you," "Medicine can work miracles nowadays," or "This will make better people of you." Often the parent suspects that these comments are designed to make the speaker, rather than the parent, feel better. The parent's sense of isolation and anger is increased.

How a parent chooses to respond to well-meaning comments or decides how much of the situation to share will depend on whether the other person in question is a relative, a close friend, or an inquisitive stranger. In the early stages, the very idea that there may be a choice of responses may seem surprising to parents. The emotions triggered by the remarks and questions of other people are so intense and so near the surface that it is difficult to discuss the child's situation with anything approaching matter-of-factness. The parents are apt to be engulfed by their feelings and to feel that there is little choice except to either turn away from the other person or to run the risk of breaking down into tears if they try to talk about it.

It does become increasingly possible to make choices between ways of responding to others. To make these choices, it is necessary to think about two major aspects of the interaction. First, who is the person who is making the comment? Is it someone the parent feels close to or has frequent contact with? Or is this a stranger the parent is unlikely to meet again? It will be much more important that the person the parent sees often has an understanding of the disability and its effects than the stranger who may be simply curious or insensitive.

Second, parents will want to consider what it is that they would like from this person. Do they want understanding and support? Acceptance of the child? Or do they wish that the person would not notice the child's problem? Knowing what the parent would like to have from another person can help in making decisions about how much effort to invest in attempting to reach an understanding with that person.

When a child is born with a disability, an issue that arises immediately is that of notifying friends and relatives of the birth. Usually, these people have known of the pregnancy and are eagerly awaiting the news. What is a new parent to do? Some new parents go ahead and fill out the prepared birth announcements, adding a note on each about the baby's situation. Others remain silent, letting the family grapevine take charge of spreading the news. Such a hit-or-miss method seems to be unfair to those who are genuinely concerned about the family. Friends and relatives may be embarrassed if they have sent bubbly and enthusiastic messages of congratulations, only to discover later that the baby has a disability. If they hear reports of grief and woe from other family members they may be uncertain as to how to approach the new parents. Hearing the news directly from the parents enables them to get a more accurate picture of what is going on and provides clues as to how they can respond.

RELATIVES

To young parents engrossed in the tasks of establishing and providing for their growing immediate family, the arrival of a child with a disability may seem to be a very private crisis. In truth, a larger family network will be deeply affected by this event. Echoes and repercussions will travel the entire length of the family tree.

The child's grandparents are often overlooked in the intensity of the immediate situation. Grandparents have their own grief and pain to deal with. They have had their own dreams of security and success for their children and grandchiildren. They may have been enjoying the freedom and satisfaction that comes from having raised children to be independent and self-sufficient. Now, they are drawn back into worrying about their children. They may feel it is necessary once again to offer financial or emotional support to their grown children.

Grandparents are often caught in another generation's ideas and attitudes about handicaps. Horror, pity, or a feeling that handicaps are God's punishment for past sins may mingle with their feelings of concern for their children. Grandparents may have a greater need to search for causes or explanations, or to look into the in-laws family for evidence that such traits did not originate in their own side of the family tree. But they may also have the perspective and the wisdom that come from having weathered difficult times in their own lives.

Grandparents need to be included in both the pains and the joys of the child's life. Indeed, they can be a powerful source of support for parents. Farber found that frequent interaction with the wife's mother was related to a higher degree of marital stability in families with children who were retarded.[1] This was found to be true regardless of the degree of dependence of the retarded child and so was interpreted by Farber to be related to emotional support rather than actual physical assistance with the child's care.

But accepting help, whether financial or emotional, from their own parents can result in a dilemma for parents of a child with a disability. The need to be independent and to provide for one's own family is very strong in young adulthood. It may be very uncomfortable for young parents to acknowledge and accept help from their own parents. Accepting such help may seem to carry with it a feeling of obligation, regardless of whether the grandparent who offers the help means it to or not.

The grandparents, aunts, and uncles of the disabled child will need to share with the parents in the grieving to be done. For, just as with parents, it is only by passing successfully through the stage of grieving that they will be able to share fully in the joy and pride in the child that follows. Children with disabilities need to be able to enjoy and benefit from relationships with other close relatives as much as, if not more than, other children. It may be difficult for some parents to cry with or express their fears to their own parents. And it may be even more difficult to try to cope with someone else's grief when one's own seems all but unmanageable. But it is not necessary to "cure" the grandparents' grief, all that is necessary is to share it. In the sharing, the bonds of love and support are strengthened.

The brothers and sisters of the parents will likewise need to share in the grieving of the family. If they are in the process of creating their own families, they may have fears or worries about whether the disability is inherited and whether they might have a child affected by it. These fears may not be voiced for fear that they will seem selfish or petty in light of the child's parents' difficulties. The parents may need to say, "You may be wondering about your chances of having a child with . . . ," and to outline what they have learned, telling their brothers and sisters where genetic counseling is available if this is appropriate.

FRIENDS

Many parents feel isolated and estranged from even their closest friends. This experience seems so painful and so overwhelming that it seems that no one else can understand. If there is one common theme in the development of parent groups throughout the country, it is, "We felt so alone."

It may be true that friends feel awkward and embarrassed because they are not sure what is the "right" thing to say. After all, they probably have not had much experience in dealing with this kind of situation. We need only to remember the first funeral we ever attended, and how we rehearsed carefully the words we would say to the bereaved, to realize how important past experience is in contributing to feeling at ease in difficult situations.

But it may be equally true that parents unwittingly contribute to creating this distance between themselves and their freinds. Parents may dread talking to their friends about the situation for a variety of reasons. In the beginning, the parent truly does not know what to expect. How will the child do? Will he or she be able to manage as a parent? Will the parent, or others, be embarrassed by the child? A flood of doubts and questions can make it difficult to talk even to those the parents are closest to.

Parents may fear that if they try to talk honestly and openly with friends, they will collapse into tears. They need to ask themselves: what would be so terrible about that? Many of us have been raised to keep a "stiff upper lip" and keep our troubles to ourselves. Tears are to be shed privately; any crying in front of others is abhorrent. And yet, the experience of sharing pain may be one of the healthiest and most healing ways to deal with that pain.

Other times, parents may feel that they do not want to be a burden to others. They may not want their friends to pity or feel sorry for them. When it is difficult to imagine feeling cheerful about anything, it may seem to the parent that the friendship will become lopsided, with the friend continually being the one offering the comfort and support. Or, they may worry that sharing too much about the child and their own fears will somehow prejudice people against the child and make them less able to accept and enjoy her.

Naturally, it is necessary for a parent to make judgments about who to talk to about the situation and how much to share. The parent may feel truly unable to say much about what he or she is experiencing but not wish to be cold or curt to a friend who is asking. In such cases, it may be sufficient to say simply, "I'm feeling pretty upset and worried right now," or "We can't do much more than wait and see right now, but I would still like to see you." "I appreciate your asking" is never inappropriate.

Good friends will appreciate a parent's honesty, even if it means just being told that the parent is not ready to talk about it. One mother reported that after she was feeling better about herself and her child she realized how she had deprived both herself and her friends of an opportunity for sharing. She said that one friend told her, "I know it was hard for you, but you made it very hard for your friends too."

Friends are not only for sharing sorrows with, they are also for having fun with. The parent who makes the effort to continue contacts and activities with friends may find that this is one way to begin to restore a more satisfying balance to his or her own life. And effort it may take, especially in the beginning. It may be very difficult to join friends for coffee or outings when one feels filled with despair or even guilt about enjoying oneself in the midst of such a tragic situation. But it is necessary to learn that other aspects of life do go on, and that it is possible to take pleasure from them once again.

Close friends who are incorporated into the situation may also prove to be valuable sources of assistance in very practical ways. A friend may be available to baby-sit on short notice so that a mother may have her hair done, shop for a few hours, or even just take a nap. Friends or relatives may need reassurance or instruction about the child's care in order to feel comfortable in taking over. Parents would do well to remember what their own fears and questions were when they learned to care for the child and use these as a basis for explaining to others what the child needs. Allowing friends and relatives who visit the home to hold, feed, and play with the child as naturally as they would with any other child will help them to feel comfortable in doing these things. It will also make it possible for these friends and relatives to experience firsthand the fun and satisfaction to be had from the child. There is no better way to achieve a natural acceptance of the child as an individual. People who can get to know a baby or child with a disability, who can laugh and play games with her, will be able to see and appreciate that child's personality and strengths. They will be more able to see the whole child and not just her disability. And *that* goal is very important to most parents.

While it is very necessary to be able to share feelings of sadness and worry, it is also important to most parents that they themselves not be viewed with pity, as though their own lives were being lived in an atmosphere of constant tragedy. This takes some time, certainly; but it also requires the opportunity to experience together some of the lighter moments.

Parents may even discover that it is possible to find humor in the child's situation. The clumsiness of orthopedic appliances and the naiveté of retardation lend themselves well to "black" jokes when the parents' own adjustment has reached the point where humor is again possible. This may be quite shocking to outsiders who expect families to be grim or tearful in the face of a disability. It is disconcerting; it does not "fit" into stereotyped expectations. Such humor can be a very healthy way to apply new definitions to unavoidable circumstances. To break the stranglehold of "This is a disaster" and to change it to include "Some parts of this are funny" is to experience new freedom in ways of reacting and being human.

It may, however, still be necessary to choose rather carefully when and with whom to share these moments. One couple reported an incident that occurred when they were hosting a small, rather elegant dinner party. Their 5-year-old daughter was upstairs in her room. From her bedroom came the familiar sounds of "thump, thump, clunk" as she walked about with her crutches. Suddenly, there was a loud crash. It was obvious that she had fallen. The host paused briefly as he poured the wine, listening for the cries which would mean that she had hurt herself. When there were none he said, blandly, "Ah, yes — we always did want to hear the pitter-patter of little feet." A stunned silence greeted his remark. Clearly, these dinner guests had not shared enough of the good times as well as the bad to be able to incorporate such an irreverant attitude into their reactions.

STRANGERS: THE WORLD OUTSIDE

It is one thing to know that one ought to continue with the activities
that are a part of everyday life, going on errands, shopping, making
trips to libraries, restaurants, and public events, and that it is desirable
to take along the infant or child with a disability whenever one would
ordinarily take a child along. It may be quite another thing to
contemplate actually being accompanied by a child who will draw
the curiosity or pity of total strangers. Suddenly, how a parent reacts
to the child or to other people's reactions will be on display. How to
deal with questions or how to explain the child's situation become
important issues.

Since babies are not expected to be able to walk or talk, many
disabilities are not immediately obvious in a very young child. When
people on the street or in shops stop to admire or coo over the baby,
parents may feel a strange compulsion to explain to total strangers all
about the kinds of problems the child has. How does one respond to
the passer-by who exclaims, "My, what a beautiful baby!"? It may
seem awkward to accept compliments from people who assume that
the child is as free of difficulties as we expect all infants to be.

It is more likely, however, that this urge to "tell all" to strangers
on the street reflects the parent's own uncertainty and mixed feelings
about the child. When the child's disability seems to be the most
striking thing about her, it is difficult for parents to think of their
baby without also thinking of the disability. The disability and the
parents' own feelings about it are in the forefront of their minds. It
is difficult to enjoy the baby's cuteness or her smile without feeling
the sadness about her situation. This mixture of emotions prompts
the parent to respond to "What a beautiful baby!" with, "Yes, but
she . . . "

Parents can take some comfort from the knowledge that the
acuteness of their conflicting feelings will subside with time. The
balance will shift as they become better acquainted with the growing
child and are able to experience more moments of pleasure both in
their relationship with the child and in their own lives.

But parents should not necessarily expect that their feelings and
responses will occur or change in orderly stages. While many of the
written descriptions of parental reactions have a great deal of validity,
an individual parent's feelings are not likely to fall into neat or clearly
defined patterns. As Betty Pieper, the mother of a teenager with
multiple disabilities, writes, ". . . I have never seen any literature which
properly described my feelings . . . My feelings continue to run the
full range, depending upon the circumstances. My feelings were not
confined to special 'stages' or a given order."[2] The ability to accept

as natural the mixture of feelings parents have, no matter how "disordered" they may seem to be, can contribute to being able to respond to others more effectively.

There is no denying that there are tactless people in the world, and that parents are bound to encounter some of them. "What's wrong with her?" can be a disconcerting question when asked unexpectedly on a bus or in a store. It can evoke a variety of responses from embarrassment to rage.

When a total stranger asks an abrupt or rude question, parents need feel under no obligation to provide a full explanation or even to be polite if they do not wish to be. It is helpful for a parent to consider what he or she wishes to accomplish in this kind of situation. Is it to educate this "ignorant" person? To explain the disability? Or is the goal to find a snappy response which will put the person "in his place"?

Factual answers can be very brief. "She is retarded" or "Her legs are paralyzed" may suffice. Gentle reproofs may be comments like, "I'd rather talk about what is *right* with her." Not-so-gentle rebukes can be limited only by one's imagination or distaste for public scenes. Exploring possible responses and the feelings these comments evoke with other parents of children with disabilities can be very helpful in arriving at a comfortable way to deal with these situations.

The situation becomes more complicated as the child grows older. Not only will the disability probably be more apparent to other people, thus attracting more notice, but the child herself may become aware of other people's curiosity and of her parent's discomfort. The child whose parents are uncomfortable or embarrassed by the attention paid to her appliances, her appearance, or her behaviors will have a difficult time learning to move about in the world with ease. If, on the other hand, the child can observe the parents responding matter-of-factly and tactfully to curious people, she too can learn to be more comfortable in public.

The parent who finds herself becoming tense or uncomfortable in public would do well to give some thought to the possible sources of discomfort. It may be that public scrutiny brings to the surface some of the "hidden" feelings about the child's disability. Feelings of guilt, shame, or anger may still be present long after we think we have "rationally" overcome them. Honestly admitting to oneself that traces of these feelings still exist is a major step in learning to deal with them in a way that is not destructive to parents themselves or to their children.

The discomfort may arise because somehow the parents feel that onlookers may think that they are not "good parents." This is especially likely if the child's behaviors seem inappropriate for her age or size or are obtrusive enough to be readily noticed. In this situation, a hard cold look at reality might help. Does it *really* matter whether the passengers on the bus think that one is a good parent or not? Even if someone did get off the bus thinking, "My, that was a terrible parent," what would the "awful" consequences be?

The world, fortunately, is changing. More and more children and adults with disabilities are taking their rightful places in the mainstream of life and are quietly going to public schools, holding jobs, and living in "ordinary" neighborhoods. Children are growing up who have had classmates with disabilities. These children will not be unduly startled or shocked by meeting people with wheelchairs or differences in speech or movement. The combined efforts of parent groups, agencies, coalitions, and adults with disabilities have had an effect on the awareness and acceptance of those who are not disabled.

In practical, everyday terms, this means that parents are less and less likely to meet people who are totally without any exposure or experience with disabilities. Strangers may look at children with disabilities for many reasons. Often, for example, a woman who is watching a child with a disability may be thinking of her cousin or her neighbor who has a child with a problem, and wondering if she dares to ask the child's parent about possible resources for her cousin or neighbor.

The world "belongs" to the child with a disability as much as it does to the rest of us. The child needs the opportunity to experience it, explore it, and learn to move about in it.

QUESTIONS FOR PARENTS

1. Can I share my feelings about my child's disability with the people who are close to me?
2. Is it possible for me to accept freely genuine offers of help when I need it?
3. Can I let people know that I appreciate their concern even when I don't want to talk about it?
4. How can I let my relatives and friends know that I also wish to continue sharing in good times and fun?
5. How can I let people know that I don't want their pity?
6. Can I allow relatives and friends to experience being with my child so they can learn to know him and enjoy her?
7. If I am uncomfortable or tense when strangers notice or comment on my child, can I identify the sources of that discomfort?
8. Do I need to "rehearse" my responses to tactless comments from strangers?

REFERENCES

1. Farber, Bernard, Effects of a Severely Mentally Retarded Child on Family Integration, *Monograph of the Society for Research in Child Development*, Vol. 24, No. 2., 1959.
2. Pieper, Betty, *When Something is Wrong with Your Baby . . . Looking In and Reaching Out*, Spina Bifida Association of America, 1977.

4
FINDING AND MAKING USE OF PROFESSIONAL HELP

Once the reality of the child's problem has been acknowledged, the question of providing for that child's special needs comes to the forefront. Unless the parent has been unable to move from the stage of denial, it will be clear that all the parent's love and acceptance will not be enough. This child will need more. He or she may need medical care and treatment, adaptations or special approaches in mobility or communication training, special education or habilitation programs, or other services.

For some families, pride in being able to meet their own needs independently is an important value. To be forced by circumstances to ask for outside help, particularly financial assistance, may be, to these families, an indication of failure or incompetence. Often, these implications are not recognized or stated explicitly. Instead, they operate below the surface to interfere with matter-of-fact discussions of the options available to meet the child's needs.

All families, however, are likely to be faced with a situation in which they must make decisions about the child's care and give consent for treatment in areas outside of their own spheres of knowledge and experience. They may be plunged into technical discussions of diagnoses and treatment plans long before they can comprehend what the child's disability means or what services are available.

Raising a child poses awesome responsibilities for any parent. The business of caring for and nurturing a young and helpless human being, instilling values, teaching skills, and, finally, allowing the child gradually to venture forth on his own is one of life's most complex and challenging tasks.

The parent of the child with a disability retains all of these responsibilities. Society may, depending on the nature of the handicap, somewhat alter or delay some of its expectations, but is still expects the parent to be responsible for some degree of socially acceptable behaviors and skills on the part of the child unless the child is totally turned over to the society (to live in an institution, for example). Thus, while the general societal goal of toilet training by about the age of 2½ years may be altered for the child with a disability, it is still expected that within a few additional years some socially acceptable system for handling body wastes will be achieved. Parents are expected to ensure that "undesirable" behaviors are curbed in public and that the child receives training in caring for himself.

In previous generations, the family was expected quietly to assume all care for its members who were "different." "Feebleminded" children or "odd" aunts or uncles lived with their families as long as they did not become too disruptive to the community. The changing patterns of American family life: increased mobility, smaller families, more frequent divorce and remarriage, and the new awareness of the human rights of persons with disabilities have changed some of this. New attitudes, new knowledge, new resources, and new programs have opened up new avenues of hope and expectations for families of children with disabilities.

As soon as the child's disability is discovered, or even as soon as the parent suspects that a disability is present and wishes to have the suspicion either confirmed or denied, the need for professional help is apparent. The parent may rapidly find himself adrift in a sea of unfamiliar terminology, conflicting opinions, and a host of bewildering agencies and programs. How is a parent to make sense of all this and make the choices best for his child?

Sometimes, decisions about treatment for the child must be made immediately after birth. This situation is fraught with pitfalls. It is difficult to imagine how parents can possibly give truly informed consent at this time. It is difficult, if not impossible, to comprehend the meaning of the disability itself at this point, and even more so to grapple with the implications of treating or not treating.

The parents are probably more dependent than they will ever be on the advice and opinions offered by the professional people involved. The parent who has never heard of the condition before, and who is all but overwhelmed by shock, has very little else to go on. The professional obligation to be possessed of the most up-to-date information possible and to keep one's own personal biases in check is never more acute.

A serious time lag exists between the development of learning through research and its wide dissemination to practitioners in all professions. In the field of social work, this lag may be more than 10 years. In medicine, the process of accumulating data, writing about the results, presenting the material at professional meetings, and finally reaching widespread dissemination through books or other publications may also take years.

In the case of a condition like spina bifida, in which immediate treatment decisions are often necessary and in which the preferred methods of treatment have changed dramatically over the last few decades, the results of this lag may be tragic. The information current during one's professional training only a few years earlier may already be outdated. Many families have been encouraged not to treat their children with spina bifida, to "let them die," on the basis of outdated information. The physician confronted with a condition outside his usual scope of practice must exercise his obligation to seek additional information or to refer the child before he issues pronouncements as to what should be done.

The fact that the ultimate responsiblity for the child, regardless of how many professionals are involved or how competent they may be, rests in the final analysis with the parent is painfully clear to most parents. Every parent who has signed his name to a "Consent for Surgery" form for his infant has had this brought home with dramatic impact.

And yet, most parents feel that their relationships with the professionals who treat their children do not reflect this responsibility. These parent-professional relationships seem unbalanced. To many parents, it seems as though the "expert" holds most of the authority and power, and the parent is expected to remain in the position of grateful recipient. It takes courage on both parts to change this traditional pattern and to forge a new kind of parent-professional relationship which recognizes the authority and responsibility of both. The professional must be able to react to questions as questions and not as challenges; and the parent must be firm in asserting his or her rights and responsibilities. Each must respect the other.

The conscientious parent will need to assure himself that he is, as far as he is able, making the best possible decisions for the child. The parent will need to learn all that he can about the disability and its treatment. Whether the help the child needs is surgical, medical, educational, or habilitative, the parent will need to make some assessments of the skill and competence of the persons delivering those services.

The professional who is not accustomed to having his judgments questioned may be taken aback by parental scrutiny not only of his decisions but of his credentials and his attitudes. The competent have nothing to fear. Indeed, the child whose parents understand, agree with, and support the treatment program and rationale is likely to do far better than the child whose parents disagree or do not understand.

It is, fortunately, easier today than it was even a few years ago to locate information written for parents about disabilities. Any parent would be well advised to contact Closer Look for information on services, resources, and issues (ask to be put on their mailing list for their free newsletter), the National Foundation–March of Dimes and the National Easter Seal Society for Crippled Children and Adults provide information on birth defects, disabilities, publications, and other organizations (see Appendix A for mailing addresses). Many voluntary groups have both national organizations and local chapters and can provide a wealth of information on specific disabilities as well as the support of being in contact with other families who live with the same problems. (See Appendix A in this book for a listing of organizations and addresses. Books and other publications are listed in Appendix B.)

The issue of determining which professional approach and which particular specialist will best meet the needs of the child is very difficult. No matter what professional background a parent may himself have, he is likely to need to call upon the services of disciplines totally unfamiliar to him. How, short of becoming a trained specialist oneself, can one hope to make intelligent choices in these other fields?

Some guidelines can be offered to parents who wish to assess whether a particular professional person is a good choice for their child, and whether the professional and the parent will be able to work together.

First and most obviously, one can inquire about the person's professional training. What degrees does the person hold? In which fields? From what universities? If the person is a medical or surgical specialist, is he Board-certified or Board-eligible in his field? While research activities are not necessarily related to good practice, if the person has been involved in research or has written publications in the field you may want to know this or to read them.

It may be important to ascertain that the person is up-to-date on current developments in the field. Does he or she attend meetings and subscribe to journals in the area of your concern? Does he or she suggest new approaches or new research findings to you? Is he or she willing to collaborate with others to share approaches and ideas?

Does the professional person keep you informed? Do you have access to information about tests and evaluations performed on your child? Is the treatment plan and its goals made clear to you, and do you have the opportunity to ask questions about it? Are alternative approaches discussed with you? Are both the expected benefits and the limitations of the planned program explained fully?

The arrangements for contact with the professional person should be specified. How often will he or she be meeting with you or your child? What procedures are to be followed if you have questions between appointments, or if unforeseen difficulties or emergencies occur? Under what circumstances does the professional person wish to be notified between regular visits?

When you are branching out into a new area of treatment or training for your child, you will want to seek recommendations from others who are knowledgeable. Is the person you are considering one of those recommended by other professionals you have worked with? Does he or she work with other children who have the same condition that your child does? You can be doubly assured of a choice when both professionals and other parents whose children are receiving those services speak favorably of a person.

Most parents will want to know something about the professional's philosophy of care and attitudes toward children and toward dissabilities. Some of this can be asked directly, while some is best determined by observing how the person relates to you and to your child. What overall approach and goals does the person have? Even in a relatively straightforward area like bracing for physical handicaps, differences of opinion exist as to the goals of bracing and the best ways to accomplish them.

Does the professional person see the child's problem in the broader perspective of the child as a whole? Does the professional show that he values that child for what he is and what he can do? Or does he or she see the child as needing to be protected? Does the orthopedic surgeon, for example, see just the dislocated hip or does he appreciate the person that that hip belongs to, the child who must, experience the pain and the confinement of surgery and who, it is hoped, will walk or sit better on that hip? Some parents have encountered professionals who have felt that a particular treatment was not "worth it" for a particular child, even though the parent wished the child to have the treatment. Such an obvious difference in values can leave a parent feeling helpless, frustrated, and enraged. Other differences in attitudes and values may be less obvious but just as destructive to a good working relationship.

The thoughtful parent knows that he or she is the person most intimately familiar with the child and the ways in which the child deals with his problem. Does the professional ask for and incorporate the parent's assessment of the child into the treatment plan? Does he or she really listen to the parent's observations of behaviors, symptoms, or abilities? Does he or she reevaluate the treatment approach when the parent reports difficulties with following through at home?

The child's well-being and progress often depend, to some extent at least, on a good working relationship between the parents and the professional people involved. The interactions may or may not be important in a particular situation. If the child needs a highly specialized surgical procedure, it is likely that the parents will want to have the best-qualified surgeon and will not care a great deal whether they like his personality or not. If, on the other hand, the situation is one in which the parents and the professional must work together over a long period of time, issues of personality may assume more importance.

The parent will probably also be concerned with how openminded the professional is. A willingness to admit to what is not known with certainty and to ask the opinions of other experts can be essential if the parent is to be able to relax and have confidence in the professional's judgment. Many parents tell me that they perceive "messages" from persons treating their children to the effect that if they go elsewhere for consultation or treatment, they "might as well not come back." Such attitudes, if they are being perceived correctly, have no place in responsible professional practice. It is doubtful that many of these people would themselves sign consent forms for their own children without seeking other opinions to assure themselves that this was the best thing to do under the circumstances.

Rarely, if ever, are these kinds of concerns and expectations made explicit by either party when a relationship is entered into by a parent and a professional. The parent might not even be aware that he holds certain expectations about the kind of treatment he wishes for his child until he perceives that something is lacking. Both parties might do well to remember that this is indeed a contractual type of agreement, with both sides having certain expectations of and obligations to the other.

The parent, too, has certain obligations and responsibilities in these partnerships. Indeed, the success of most activities and treatment programs depends upon parental understanding and support. Most treatments, be they medical or educational, are not simply "done to" a child in a clinic or school setting. They have implications and repercussions at home as well. A child who is retarded and who is being taught skills in feeding, dressing, or communication may be baffled or confused if different methods are used at home. Medical and surgical treatments often require that medications, exercises, or observation of symptoms be continued at home for long periods of time.

The parent shares with the professional person the responsibility for making sure that the goals of the treatment or intervention are clear to both and that the part each will play is understood. If a

surgical procedure is being contemplated, exactly what is it designed
to accomplish? Which aspects of the child's problem will it affect, and
which will it not? How will it affect the child's care or routine at
home? If an educational or training program is to be instituted, exactly
how is the parent to follow through at home?

Often the actual time that the parent and the professional person
spend together is very short. The demands of a busy office or clinic
may not lend themselves to lengthy, relaxed discussions. When the
parent must also keep an eye on a squirming, restless, or frightened
child, he or she may find it especially difficult to concentrate on
ensuring that all of the issues are addressed.

The parent can help to insure that this time is used to accomplish
what the parent wants by having his concerns and questions clearly
in mind prior to the appointment. Most parents find it necessary and
useful to bring in writing any questions that they have as well as a
summary of any observations they have made that they wish to bring
to the professional's attention.

Jotting down the key points covered in the discussion is helpful
also. When we are anxious or distracted we may find it difficult to
recall exactly what was said. If one parent is not present at the child's
appointment, the notes may help the parent who was there to
remember all the points covered so that both are informed. If the
parent feels that the time was too short, or if he has questions that he
is uncomfortable in raising in front of the child, he should request
another appointment, making it clear that he desires time for a more
complete discussion of the issues in the situation. This is often useful
periodically to be sure that the working parent who, because of work
schedules, is often not present during routine appointments is brought
up to date and has his or her own opportunity to ask questions and
voice concerns. These joint meetings will also relieve the parent who
usually does take the child to appointments (most often, this is still
the mother) from the uncomfortable responsibility for explaining or
justifying treatment approaches to the other parent. Both parents are
then more free to question and to share more equally in the decisions
about approaches for the child.

The relationship between parent and professional carries with it
the responsibility for a certain amount of honesty and candor on both
sides. The professional is expected to call upon his knowledge, training,
and skills and to share with the parents his assessment of how these can
best be utilized for the benefit of the child.

The parent, however, bears the ultimate responsibility for the
child's welfare. He or she must give written consent for surgical
procedures and must also indicate agreement with the Individualized
Education Plan formulated for the child who is to receive special

education services. The parent is responsible for asking questions about the proposed treatment programs and for contributing his or her own knowledge about the child's personality, abilities, and reactions.

It is important for the parent to voice his concerns about proposed programs for the child or about goals or implementation of programs already underway. Much of the time, this will result in a better understanding of the plans and activities on behalf of the child.

Sometimes, however, the ensuing discussion will reveal that the parent still has reservations about or even disagreement with the recommendations. This presents a new problem for the parent. He may wish to consider seeking additional opinions or evaluations of his child, or to investigate alternative programs. However, the parent will be in a better position to assess the situation and take constructive action rather than remaining bewildered or resentful about the child's treatment.

Questioning what is done for one's child can be an uncomfortable thing to do for many parents for a variety of reasons. Most of the time, programs for the child fall outside the area of the parents' own expertise, and the lack of knowledge of the specific field can leave them feeling at a disadvantage. White coats, fancy offices, and titles such as M.D. or Ph.D. can still be intimidating to parents who may have had less education.

Many parents will tend to hold back on their concerns or criticisms for another reason. Parents are acutely aware of what happens in professional circles when a client, a patient, or a family is labeled as being "difficult." Parents do not wish to be labeled as "problems," for fear that their genuine concerns might be discounted, or, even worse, that their child might somehow be slighted. Barsch agrees that parents have been unduly stigmatized by being labeled as "anxiety-ridden," "overprotective," or "guilt-ridden."[1] Those of us who have been on both sides of this particular fence recognize that these fears are not totally unjustified.

Parents do have a responsibility to try to see that their concerns are expressed directly and to the point. It can be very difficult to keep other emotions — anger about the disability in general or about a previous treatment, or anxiety about the expense of a program or the ultimate outcome for the child — from influencing how one reacts to a situation concerning the child. An awareness of this can help to keep questions about the child's treatment from erupting as attacks on the professionals.

Often it is appropriate and helpful to obtain a second or even a third opinion on the child's disability or on a proposed treatment program. Both courtesy and practicality dictate that the parent notify the person who is treating the child that he wishes to consult with someone else. The professional may have suggestions for people the parents might wish to seek opinions from. Often, test results or x-rays can be copied and taken to the consultant to avoid the expense, time, and possible risks of unnecessary repetition.

The parent has a responsibility to be both accurate and honest in reporting back to the professional on aspects of the program carried out at home. Exercises, medications, or other activities may be prescribed for specific amounts of time, and the professional will need to know to what extent the family found it possible to follow his or her recommendations in order to assess whether the program is worthwhile or whether it needs to be altered.

Many disabling conditions require that the child receive services from a variety of specialized areas. In spina bifida, to name but one example, the child will ordinarily need treatment and monitoring by a neurosurgeon, urologist, orthopedist, orthotist, and pediatrician; and may also need the services of physical and occupational therapists, psychologists, social workers, and special educators. The child's care may become fragmented, with each specialist working diligently on his or her "piece" of the child but with no one clearly in charge of the overall situation. Sometimes, plans and treatment programs may actually conflict with each other if the professionals are not in communication with each other; or the child and his family may be overburdened by instructions for at-home care and management coming from many different sources at once.

Whose job shall it be to assess the child's total situation and to make judgments about what kinds of interventions are needed at what points in the child's life? The parent's? The pediatrician's? The specialist who is most actively involved at this particular time? The social worker's? Often, this task seems to fall by default to the parent. This can sometimes be quite workable if the parent feels comfortable with it and feels that he has the knowledge he needs to know when the child needs a particular kind of help and where at least to begin looking for it. But it can be quite uncomfortable, too, when it means constantly keeping track of when follow-ups and tests are due or anxiety about whether all that should be done is being done.

The fragmentation of care that can result from our system, with many agencies and individuals treating a child, can thus present a serious problem that is difficult for parents to deal with. How is a parent to know which resource he should be looking for? How does he learn where services are located? How does he know that something important is not being overlooked?

Brewer and Kakalik, reporting on a Rand Corporation study done for the Department of Health, Education, and Welfare, write that information about available services and direction to an appropriate mix of services is severely lacking in this country. Further, they find that the range of services available within a reasonable distance of the family home is often incomplete.[2] Some parents eventually learn that better services are available in a different geographical area and face difficult choices about whether to move the family for the child's sake. Brewer and Kakalik recommend the establishment of regional direction centers, which could be utilized by parents to guide them to the services their children need.

Until such resources exist, what can a parent do? The first step is to recognize the need for someone to oversee and evaluate the child's needs as he develops. This person must be familiar with the particular disability and the problems it presents, the current recommended treatment for those problems, and the availability of resources in the particular city and state. Sometimes, it can be the pediatrician who already knows the family and who is willing to keep abreast of the disability and the specialized treatment it requires. Sometimes it can be the coordinator of the clinic where the child receives services. Other times, it can be a specialist who is knowledgeable about the overall situation and whom the parents trust. Meetings and newsletters of groups of the disabled and their parents can be valuable sources of information for parents on services available in the area.

Regardless of who the parents decide can best fulfill this role, it is absolutely imperative that a frank and explicit discussion be held about what this role involves and what each expects from this type of relationship. It simply is not safe to assume that someone is doing this if in fact an explicit agreement has not been reached.

Much of the preceding discussion has made it sound as though parents do in fact have many choices about the treatment that the child receives. Often, this is simply not true. As Brewer and Kakalik state, "our society operates on the pervasive but erroneous assumption that the parents of handicapped children, like any other consumers, have unrestricted choices about the services they obtain for their children."[2] In many cases, this is a myth. All services are not equally distributed to all geographical areas of this country. There may be only one treatment center anywhere near within a reasonable traveling distance for a particular problem, or, even worse, there may be none. Or, there may be restrictions attached to financial assistance as to where the treatment may be obtained. Is there anything that families in these situations can do, short of uprooting the entire family to move to another city, or hoping that a rich uncle on his deathbed will be discovered in the family tree?

The first thing that a parent in this kind of dilemma can do is to be sure that in fact the choices do not exist. This means collecting information on what services do exist in the area. Often, this information has already been collected by someone else. Information, referral, or directory services or listings may be available from city or municipal departments, health and social agencies, voluntary organizations, or groups and coalitions for and of the disabled. Meeting and talking with other consumers — other parents and adults with disabilities — can also yield important information.

If the problem seems to be that a third party that pays for all or part of the services (the state, for example) has restrictions on where those services can be obtained, the parent should be sure not to accept someone else's word for this. The parent needs to go directly to the people in charge of such authorizations, explain what services are desired and from whom, and ask for clarification of the policies on this. Some states that provide assistance for children with disabilities, for example, are willing to pay for services rendered in an adjoining state while others are not.

Even if a parent is, by practical considerations, limited to a particular institution or program, there are legitimate and useful ways to approach the problem of dissatisfactions with that program.

If the problem seems to be that the parent has doubts about the wisdom of following the recommendations offered for the child, the question may be clarified by seeking another opinion in a tactful but open way, without cutting the child off from the services he is currently receiving. For some families, paying for the cost of a one-shot consultation with a top expert in a neighboring state may well be worth the expense in terms of the peace of mind it brings. If the consultant agrees with the treatment the child is currently receiving, the parent will be able to relax and enjoy more confidence in the people who are caring for the child.

If the consultant disagrees with the current program, the parent is in a more difficult situation. At the very least, the situation has been clarified to the extent that the differences of opinion are out in the open. Perhaps a frank and open discussion of the approaches and treatment with the people currently involved can help the parent to see the rationale and the reasons behind the differing approaches. If this discussion can remain focussed on approaches the child's needs and be kept free of anger from the parent and defensiveness on the part of the professional, a solution may be possible. The professional may even be stimulated to increase his or her own knowledge by learning more about new or alternative approaches to the problem.

Perhaps the parent feels that the problem he sees with services is one other parents are also experiencing or is related to the way in which the services are delivered. In such a case, it may well be possible to work with other parents and within the system to effect changes. The first step in this case is to learn whether other parents are experiencing the same difficulties, by talking with them, calling them on the telephone, or setting up a meeting of parents involved in the program. Information collected, assembled, and written up in a dispassionate, matter-of-fact manner may stand a better chance of being taken seriously by the people in charge of the system. Such an approach also frees the parent from having to plead for his own child's case, or from the risk of being labeled a "troublemaker."

Perhaps an ally can be found in the system. This may be anyone (social worker, clinic coordinator, nurse, doctor, etc.) who is sympathetic to the problems experienced by parents and who is familiar with the mode of operation of the system involved. Such a person can often provide helpful advice on how best to present the grievances and concerns for the best chance of success. Sometimes, a formal and permanent mechanism for assuring a communication linkage between the consumers and the administrators can be built into the system. This may take the form of a Parents' Advisory Committee, for example.

One problem frequently faced by parents whose children receive care in university and training centers is that of frequent changes of personnel as trainees are rotated through the particular clinic or service. Just as the parent and child get to know a resident or other person providing care, they are confronted with yet another new face at the next appointment. Parents feel frustrated and short-changed when they must explain again and again the history of the child's problem and past treatment and how he reacts to different approaches.

While it may not be possible for parents to revise totally such a system, it may be quite possible to prod the system into adopting changes which will ameliorate these difficulties and improve the continuity of care. Some of these include the following.

1. Appointing a coordinator of care. This person can help to see that families and children receive the range of services they need from the system and that "pieces" of the child's needs are not lost. He or she can also be a central communication channel between families and the system. It is important that parents have available, and know about, a specific person to whom questions, complaints and grievances can be directed.

2. Holding more team conferences. It is vital, whenever many individual professionals are involved in a child's care, that information and treatment goals are shared with all of the people involved. Parents need to be a part of these too, so that their insights and knowledge of the child are taken into account and so that they know and understand the approaches being taken to the problem.

3. Improving record-keeping of assessments, treatment, and plans so that information is not lost. New personnel, as well as children and parents, are at a real disadvantage if summaries of previous examinations and responses to treatment programs are not readily and clearly available. Staff members who leave a service with their knowledge of a child and his family in their heads do a real disservice to their clients.

4. Improving communication between outgoing and incoming personnel. Too often, one group of trainees leaves on Friday afternoon and a new group comes in on Monday morning without any opportunity for the two groups to sit down together to share information. Such losses will not happen if meetings are formally scheduled and built into the system.

5. Increasing the educational content of the service. Seminars, conferences, guest speakers, and films can be used to educate incoming personnel about the specific conditions they will be dealing with on a particular unit or service. A solid understanding is necessary so that the staff may have a better idea of when a particular child fits or does not fit the usual patterns.

Some problems cannot be solved from within an individual service, program, or institution; they are part of the larger system of delivery of services. Programs not available in a particular area, services inadequate for the number of children who need them, or lack of availability of funds for parents to be able to make use of services are all examples of problems that call for an approach on a different level. Here parents need to look at the community and the state as a whole, and to utilize methods for bringing about social and political change. Public education about the needs of children, joining forces with advocacy groups and coalitions, and working with the legislative process are among the ways to tackle these situations (see Chapter XI).

By the time a parent has educated himself about the child's needs, has learned by trial and error how to seek out the services he wants, and has learned how to fight for the best for his child, a new, and often unexpected, issue arises. The process is often so frustrating, so painful, and so full of anxiety for the parent (lest the child suffer or be harmed from not receiving a treatment that he ought to have), that it becomes almost impossible for a parent to relax and turn over some of the responsibility for the child's care once he has found good services for the child. It is necessary for the parent to "let go" somewhat; to allow the professional to use his judgment and skills and to allow the parent to pay some attention to the direction of his own life.

This does not mean that the parent abdicates his overall responsibility for the child, but it does mean that he is not constantly on "red alert," and constantly second-guessing every decision that is made for the child. This balance between the necessary monitoring and providing for the child's needs and ensuring that a parent's own life (and that of the family) is fully lived is very difficult to achieve, but very necessary if the parent is to find the peace of mind that allows him not to sacrifice his own life for that of the child.

Parents who wish to have more children but who fear that the birth defect of condition might recur will want to obtain as much information about the disability and its causes as possible, particularly if the condition is known to have a genetic component. Local physicians or the state Department of Health may be able to provide information about genetic counseling services available in their area, as are many local branches of parent groups. The National Foundation-March of Dimes and the National Genetics Foundation (see Appendix A for addresses) may also be able to help direct parents to resources for these services.

Decisions about future pregnancies are difficult enough by themselves; without accurate information on the level of risk involved they can be overwhelming. Some birth defects can be identified (or ruled out) by tests done during pregnancy. Parents will need to learn about the tests available. It is as important to understand what the tests *cannot* do as what they can. Parents who choose testing when it is available and who receive a negative result can enjoy greater peace of mind for the remainder of the pregnancy. Parents who receive positive results, or confirmation that the birth defect is again present, can weigh that information in deciding about continuing the pregnancy or they can use it to make both psychological and practical plans for the child's birth and care.

Research into prenatal detection is continuing. For example, a new development in the case of neural tube defects (including spina bifida) involves a screening possible by testing the pregnant mother's blood. Here again, however, complete information is essential. "Positive" results on this test (called the alpha-fetoprotein, or AFP test) may be caused by a number of factors, some of them quite harmless. A positive result, therefore, simply means that more investigation is needed. This includes: a repeated blood test, rechecking of the date of the beginning of the pregnancy, and, if these are still positive, ultrasound "pictures" of the fetus and amniocentesis (the removal of a small portion of the amniotic fluid from the womb). Even a positive result at this point, however, may not be able to yield complete information on the degree of disability which will be present.

Thus there are few easy answers to questions about future children. The best that parents can do is to weigh their own

convictions and wishes along with the most complete information
they can find.

QUESTIONS FOR PARENTS

1. Do I feel that I have been told the "whole truth"?
2. If not, what do I still need to know?
3. Have I been told what my child's strengths are as well as his or
   her weaknesses?
4. Do I feel angry about the way I have been treated?
5. Am I clear about what my child needs in the immediate future?
6. Do I have some idea what his or her needs for care and treatment
   are over a longer period of time?
7. Can I ask about the things I am still uncertain about?
8. Would I like a second opinion on the diagnosis and/or treatment
   recommendations?
9. Can I let myself ask the unspoken questions about the fears I
   have for the future?
10. Do I feel that I am listened to?
11. If I have tried to ask my questions calmly of the people caring
    for my child and I have not been satisfied with the response, can
    I state again that I have unanswered questions?
12. Or do I need to consider looking for someone else to work with
    my child?
13. Does my child have a specific person responsible for coordinating
    his or her care? Or do I seem to have to do this?
14. If I feel angry about my child's care, can I make a distinction
    between that and my general anger at the unfairness of his or her
    condition?
15. Are there efforts underway in my town or city to improve services
    for children that I may consider helping with?

REFERENCES

1. Barsch, Ray., *The Parent of the Handicapped Child: The Study of
   Child-Rearing Practices*, Charles C. Thomas, 1969.
2. Brewer, Garry D. and Kakalik, James S., *Handicapped Children:
   Strategies for Improving Services*, McGraw-Hill, 1979.

5
ISSUES OF INFANCY

The needs of the young infant with a disability are much the same as the basic needs of any newborn. Food, love, security, and sleep are as important to babies with disabilities as to babies who are "normal." While it is of course true that some newborns also require medical or surgical treatment for their disabilities, many do not. In many cases, the impact of the disability is apparent not in the child but in the parents. It is the parents who are dealing with worry, grief, and shock. The newborn knows nothing of these things.

The period of infancy can be a very positive time for the entire family. Any family must go through a period of readjustment as each newborn is added to the household and its routines. Parents discover that each child's personality is different from that of her brothers and sisters. In this gradual unfolding of the unique responses and characteristics of the child with a disability lies the potential for easing the acute grief of the parents. The process of becoming acquainted with this child as a unique individual allows the parent to begin to respond to the child as a person, not as a tragedy. As the parents learn how best to satisfy the baby's needs, and see the child responding with relaxation, smiles, or contented sounds, they begin to realize that life for this child need not be all deprivation; joys and satisfactions are possible too.

Yet the early weeks and months of the child's life may also be very difficult. The child's needs do not wait for the parents to come to terms with the situation. The parents may be faced with the 24-hour-a-day round of feeding, diapering, and caring for the child at the same time that their own reactions are most acute. Fortunately, the newborn may not be aware of a parent's sorrow, although overt tension may be communicated to even the youngest of infants.

When the baby is brought home from the hospital for the first
time, parents must deal with their own uncertainties about being able
to provide the necessary care. If this child is the first-born, the parents
do not have the experience of having coped successfully with handling,
feeding, and caring for a young baby. Most first time parents, when
confronted with a seemingly totally helpless newborn, worry that the
child will choke, or be stuck with diaper pins, or that they will drop
her. These kinds of fears are apt to be exaggerated in the parents of
a child who needs special care. Parents may fear that they will be
unable to distinguish between the crying of normal "colic" and real
sickness.

When the child has required specialized medical or nursing care
in the hospital the parents' sense of competence may be further
weakened. Klaus and Kennell state that mothers who stand on the
periphery watching nurses provide care for their infants may even feel
that they are dangerous to their children.[1] Thus the words, "Your
baby is ready to go home now" can cause as much fear as relief.

It is essential that new parents have the opportunity, while the
baby is still in the hospital, gradually to take over more and more of
the care and feeding while the hospital staff remains available for
reassurance. This is important not only for the development of a
real relationship between parent and child, but in order for the parent
to have the experience of successfully meeting the child's needs. The
knowledge of their ability to cope grows with the parents' increasing
comfort in managing the care of the infant.

The parents of the baby who needs special attention to positioning,
skin care, or adaptations in feeding need careful and supportive
instructions with ample time to practice and to ask questions. These
instructions cannot be given just once; the doubts and questions may
not surface in the parent's mind until later. The parent's level of
tension may interfere with the ability to comprehend fully what is
being taught. When the child has a medical problem, the parents
need clearly to understand what signs and symptoms they should be
alert for, and under what conditions they are to call the doctor or
clinic. All instructions for care and observations should be given to
the parent in writing, along with information about who to call and
when. Parents need to know that they can call for guidance when
they are in doubt without being disparaged as panicky or overprotective.

It is a good idea for parents to begin to keep written records as
soon as the child is brought home. These records should contain both
problems and progress. The age at which the child learned to roll
over, sit up, or speak her first word may be helpful to know when she
is being evaluated later on. Parents are often amazed in later years to
discover that they cannot remember details about when particular

surgery was done, when at the time it seemed that it would be indelibly imprinted on their memories. Our memories do tend to blur details over time — sometimes, mercifully so — and it is helpful to have such a written record to retrieve needed facts quickly and accurately.

Although the basic needs of infants are similar regardless of whether or not they have disabilities, some disabilities do present special requirements or the need for adaptations in care even in infancy. Feeding, bathing, positioning, and play experiences may require special planning. While the following discussion contains general suggestions that may or may not be useful with any particular child, the parents should of course obtain specific guidance from the child's doctors or other members of the treatment team before using procedures suggested here or in any other material written for parents.

POSITIONING

The infant who has problems with his or her muscles — paralysis, lack of muscle tone, or spastic movements — may need extra attention paid to how he or she is positioned. Some of the terms used to describe problems of this type that parents may encounter are:

Spasticity: the tendency to become stiff when certain movements (such as bending the head, or straightening arms or legs) are attempted
Athetosis: uncontrolled movements of the head, arms, or legs
Hypotonia: decreased or weak muscle strength

Some children may have combinations of these.

The baby who cannot move her legs needs to be positioned so that there are no areas of pressure on the legs and they are not apt to be injured by being caught in crib slats or stroller wheels, because the skin in areas that lack normal nerve functioning is vulnerable to sores caused by pressure. The baby will not feel the pain or discomfort which would ordinarily cause her to move her legs to another position. It is for this reason that parents and babysitters need to be especially alert to the prevention of burns by protecting the skin from radiators, too-hot bath water, direct sunlight, and the like. The skin should be examined several times a day (during diaper changes is a natural time) for reddened areas that might lead to skin breakdown. If such areas are noticed, the source of the irritation must be eliminated. If the skin does break down, it will need to be kept clean, dry, and protected from further injury while it heals. Any sore that does not show steady progress in healing or that looks as if it might be infected should be brought to the attention of the child's doctor.

The child who lacks muscle tone or is "floppy" in the back, shoulders, or neck will need extra support in sitting. When the baby is small, the usual slanted infant seats may be sufficient. Sometimes the addition of small rolled-up baby blankets or towels may be used to keep the baby from slipping sideways. As the child grows to the age when she should be sitting in different places (on the floor, in high chairs, in car seats, etc.) in order to see the world about, more ingenuity may be called for. Cardboard boxes, bolsters, pieces of foam rubber, and Velcro strips are excellent, low-cost materials for constructing means of support. For practical suggestions and sketches of ways to provide extra support with inexpensive materials, the reader is referred to *Helping the Severely Handicapped Child: A Guide for Parents and Teachers.*[2]

In some conditions, such as cerebral palsy, the problem is that sets of muscles that normally act to "balance out" so that body parts remain in the position we choose are unbalanced or erratic so that parts of the body move uncontrollably or tend to be pulled into off-center positions. Another excellent resource for parents whose children have problems of this type is Nancie Finnie's *Handling the Young Cerebral Palsied Child at Home.*[3]

This book contains an excellent description of how we use sets of muscles to move, which can help parents to understand the sequences of movements necessary for their children. For example, if we wish to go from lying on our backs on the floor to a sitting position, we first have to lift our heads, then round our backs and put our arms forward. Only then can we bend our hips to complete the action.

This bending of the shoulders, neck, or hips is often necessary to enable the child with spasticity to move or be moved. If a child's arms and legs tend to be stiff, she can often be helped to relax when she is picked up if she is positioned on her side and gathered into a ball with the hips and knees bent and shoulders rounded.

The head must be centered over the midline of the body for most positions to be maintained or movements to take place. Often, the key to correct positioning of the head lies in the position of the shoulders. For example, if the child with spasticity sleeps on her back with her head extending backward, forcing itself into the pillow, she will need to have the shoulders rounded before the head and neck can assume a more normal position.

The child who tends to be stiff can often be helped in sitting or standing by being provided with a wider base of support. In a sitting position, pillows can be used to keep the legs separated. The knees should be bent with the feet supported comfortably. Both of the books mentioned above provide many other suggestions on positioning and counteracting stiff limbs in order to change a child's clothing.

FEEDING

Food is one of the most compelling needs of the young baby. One has only to observe a baby crying for food to recognize that her hunger is an all-enveloping force. Her entire body reacts with urgency to the discomfort of her stomach. The provision of food and the ensuing contented satisfaction of the baby represent warm and rewarding moments for new parents. They can feel competent to meet their child's needs, and experience warmth and tenderness in response to the baby's relaxation.

Thus problems with feeding in a young child may be especially frustrating and frightening to new parents. Worries that a baby will not get proper nourishment or that she may choke may make a parent feel tense, helpless, and inadequate. Parents may need to plan to allow feeding times to be as relaxed as possible. If the child is to be held, the parent himself needs to be seated comfortably, with his own arm supported so that it may hold the baby in a rounded yet supported manner. The use of an infant seat allows for both support of the baby and face-to-face contact with the parent. The food needs to be at the proper temperature and the right equipment assembled before beginning. Nipple holes can be enlarged or "Preemie" nipples purchased for the baby with a weak suck.

As the child progresses to sitting in a high chair, some adaptations may be necessary to enable her to sit properly. The feet should be supported, and pillows or rolled up towels can be used to keep her legs apart or to help round or support her shoulders. A low feeding chair with a larger tray may be useful for both eating and playing for a child who has difficulty in controlling movements. If belts or straps are used to help keep a child in the proper position, they should be placed over the hips and not over the soft parts of the abdomen. Parents may find additional suggestions for seats and high chairs for eating in *Parents on the Team.*[4]

As the child progresses to eating solid foods, problems with control of the jaw, tongue, and biting reflex (as in some children with cerebral palsy) may call for special techniques to be used in feeding. Parents of children with these kinds of problems should consult with their child's doctors or therapists for guidance in feeding techniques. *Helping the Severely Handicapped Child*[2] contains excellent suggestions for dealing with these situations as well as sketches illustrating ways to help the child.

Some children have difficulty in keeping their tongues in their mouths when they are eating. A reflex action acts to push the tongue forward and out of the mouth. Attempts to spoon-feed when the tongue is out of the mouth will not be successful. Parents can use a rubber-coated spoon without food on it to "walk" the tongue back in the mouth before inserting the spoon with food on it. Sometimes, pressing down on the center of the tongue with the spoon as the food is inserted can help the tongue to remain in the mouth. It may also be helpful to insert the food into the mouth along the side rather than directly in the center.

If the child tends to bite down on the spoon when it is inserted, parents can try rubbing the gums along the sides before beginning the feeding. Since this reflex can be triggered by a metal spoon touching the teeth, the use of a softer or smaller spoon may help. Parents may need to use one hand to help support the child's jaw when she is eating from a spoon or learning to drink from a cup. When facing the child, one would put the thumb under the child's chin and the forefinger on her cheek. If the parent holds the child, these positions would be reversed (i.e., the thumb would be on the cheek and the forefinger under the chin).

Eating should be a naturally enjoyable experience for the child and the parent. Mealtimes that deteriorate into anger or tension are unpleasant for both and may lead to eating problems or power struggles over food. Parents can plan for the inevitable messes by using wide trays, washable surfaces, and large bibs with pockets to collect crumbs and spills. While the use of treats or snacks need not be avoided, bottles or food should not be used to routinely "pacify" an irritable or bored child. A baby or young child who is offered food every time she cries or complains may have difficulty in learning correctly to distinguish the sensation of hunger from other tensions or discomforts, a common root of obesity in later life.

BATHING

Bathtime is, like mealtime, an excellent opportunity for parent and child to experience each other, and to talk and make sounds together. The very young baby usually needs few modifications in the usual bath routines. Parents are normally careful to check bathwater temperature and provide support for the baby's shoulders and neck with one hand while washing with the other.

Infant bathtubs that can be used on a countertop are available in most baby departments. Some of these provide some support, leaving the parent's hands more free. As the baby grows, these can also be used in a regular bathtub by cutting holes in the bottom for the circulation of water. Holes can also be cut for the insertion of straps if necessary. Also available in baby departments are plastic seats with suction cups on the bottom and a strap that goes around the baby's chest.

The times during and immediately after baths, when a baby is free of clothing and wriggling, are natural times to incorporate exercises of arms and legs. These can be transformed into games by a resourceful parent by using nursery rhymes or counting songs such as "This little piggy." The more the parent can incorporate prescribed exercises, activities, and routines into normally pleasurable events which are already a part of the family's life, the less he or she will feel burdened and restricted by the "extra" care that the child requires.

PLAY EXPERIENCES

Play experiences are not just "play" for babies and young children. Through playful experimentation with the people who care for her, by watching faces and responding with cooing sounds, the baby learns to pay attention to stimuli around her and begins to discover the satisfaction in relating warmly to another human being. This is very serious business for the infant: it is well-known that babies will fail to thrive and even die without human contact even if all their other needs are met.

This kind of learning requires frequent, close face-to-face contact. The mother (or father) who is too consumed by his or her own internal pain to be able to respond to the child, or who feels that the child is ugly or repulsive, will have difficulty with this and may need help. Such a parent needs support and understanding of the fact that these feelings are very human reactions. He or she may also need the experience of seeing someone else be able to respond to the child in a warm and positive way. Fortunately, it is often precisely when the child begins to show some response to the parent, a smile or a coo, that the parent is able to begin to perceive the child as a person and to respond himself. Thus each response of the parent or child triggers a further response in the other, and the relationship can begin to grow and build on itself.

The growing baby has needs for increasing amounts of play and stimulation. She needs to be in different rooms, to see the world from different vantage points, to experience sights, sounds, textures, and a variety of things she can handle and play with. If the child cannot do the things that other children do because of her disabilities — if she cannot crawl about, or begin to walk or talk at about the same ages as other children do — the parents will need to think about what is usual for her age and how they can best approximate those experiences.

For example, babies at 9 or 10 months of age are ordinarily crawling about and getting into much "mischief" in cupboards and closets. The baby whose legs are paralyzed can utilize a commercially made toy or just a piece of plywood on casters to move herself around the house. Parents can place her in Mommy's closet to explore her shoes while they are dressing, or put her next to the cupboard with pots and pans while they are cooking. Since babies and toddlers use their fingers to handle, manipulate, and learn about objects, the child needs ample time positioned so that his arms and fingers are not being used to support her weight and she can use them for this important "play." A bolster propped under the chest while the child is on her tummy can help support the head and chest and leave the arms more free for play.

Children need a variety of things to manipulate and play with. These need not be expensive toys. Carefully chosen inexpensive, basic toys in a variety of shapes and colors can be supplemented by objects found around the house which can be safe and interesting to a curious baby. Pots and pans, plastic utensils, flour and water, and sand are but a few examples that can be found around the house and used at the appropriate ages. Most parents find these eventually in desperation when they are stuck at home on a snowy day or the baby is cranky, but this does not lessen their usefulness.

The child who shows little interest in moving herself about should have brightly colored and interesting toys placed just out of reach so she will be motivated to get them. If she has trouble supporting herself while sitting, she needs to be propped against a couch or in her own home-made cardboard box support so that she can see the world from an upright position and have her arms and hands free for play. Some parents find that beanbag chairs are useful because they can be molded somewhat to fit the child.

It may take a very deliberate, conscious effort for parents to think about and provide these simple experiences for a child, especially if the child tends to be passive. The parent who is depressed, or who has a busy household with other active children may almost welcome immobility or passivity. However, it must be remembered that children learn by experiencing and that the more they can experience the kinds of things that other children do to grow and learn, the less they will need to make up for later. Indeed, some kinds of learning may be difficult to catch up with fully if the stage of development when the child is "ripe" for this type of learning has passed. This is not to imply that parents need to, or should, spend all their waking hours "stimulating" or "teaching" their children. It means, rather, that parents give some thought to what a child might ordinarily be doing at that particular stage of development and seek to encourage those activities in the same proportion they would expect for other children.

SPEECH DEVELOPMENT

The beginnings of speech occur early in infancy, as the baby experiments with vocal sounds when she is happy and contented. The typical times for this are when she has just been fed and is comfortable. As these early efforts are rewarded by responses from others, she is encouraged to try to do more.

The principles of helping a young child with speech difficulties are much the same as for any child who is learning to talk. As described by Nancie Finnie,[2] they are:

1. Listen to your child's sounds and early words. Show him that you hear him and will respond.
2. Be patient with his efforts. If the child can obtain what he wants with a gesture or a grunt, he will have less motivation to use words.
3. Use "real" language, not baby talk. Since this is what most parents want their children eventually to use, they must encourage it by using it themselves.
4. Repeat new sounds he has learned to make with him. Show him your pleasure in his mastery of the new sound.
5. If the child cannot talk, he needs to hear the parent talking anyway. A running commentary on what you are doing will provide needed contact and stimulation and may answer some of the questions he is unable to ask.

If the development of speech is or is expected to be a problem area for the child, parents should investigate with a speech therapist ways in which help for the child can be "built in" to the talking and communicating which is already going on between parent and child. The child may, of course, also benefit from sessions with the speech therapist. In this area it is particularly helpful for parents to work closely with the child's therapist to be as consistent as possible so that the child may, as soon as possible, be able to communicate her thoughts and ideas to the rest of her family.

HOSPITALIZATIONS

One of the most difficult tasks for the parent of a baby or very young child with a disability is to take the child to a hospital for treatment or surgery. Even though the parents may fully understand and agree that the treatment is in the child's best interest, they also know that it will be frightening and painful for the child. And no words can explain to a baby or toddler what will happen or how long she will be in this strange place.

Parents are caught in a bind. On the one hand, they must be the ones to "deliver up" the child to the hospital personnel for the treatment and to give their written consent for any procedures which are to be done. On the other, they must also provide all the comfort they can to help the child through the experience. Parents feel trapped by unacceptable alternatives; either they allow the child to receive the treatment, thus causing pain, or they do not give her the treatment and her condition worsens. Anytime people feel that they have no choices, or that the only choices they have are equally unacceptable, they are likely to feel angry, helpless, and depressed.

To make matters even worse, often very young children are perfectly aware that it is their parents who have brought them to this terrible place and are refusing to take them home. Thus they direct their anger and rage at the parents, blocking some of the comforting that is possible and arousing guilt in the parents.

The hospitalization of an infant or young child represents a severe stress for the entire family. Other children in the family feel upset and angry about their parents' absences and tensions and may have their own fears about what will happen to their brother or sister. If they are young enough, they may even fear that they too will be sent to the hospital if they are not "good" enough. These times of crisis are not times to be unnecessarily stoical and independent. Rather, there are times when help is realistically needed and should be accepted.

Fortunately, most children's hospitals and pediatric units now recognize the young child's need for the presence of her parents and not only permit but encourage parents to stay as much of the time as they can or wish. This is a far cry from the days when parents' visiting was severely restricted to "protect" the child from being upset when the parents left.

However, there still may be vexing practical problems to overcome quite apart from the worries about how the bills will be paid. If the child is hospitalized in another city, parents may need a place to sleep and rest up at intervals or for one spouse to use for sleeping while the other is at the hospital. Some hospitals will help with suggestions for low-cost rooming houses nearby. In some cities, special houses for out-of-town parents have purchased and maintained with help from McDonald's (of hamburger fame). These "McDonald Houses" offer clean, convenient rooms and an opportunity to relax with other parents and cook one's own meals at low cost. If no such help is available from the hospital staff (and parents should be sure to ask more than one person or department, since not every hospital employee will know what is available for special needs), parents can ask to talk to the social worker for suggestions or they can try calling the local parents' associations for help. Sometimes, there are parents in a city who understand and are willing to provide a spare bed to another parent who needs it.

If there are other children at home, help will be needed there too. This is not a time to be reticent about accepting offers of help from grandparents or neighbors who are familiar with the other children. Parents should, as much as is possible, explain what is expected in terms that can be understood to the child's brothers and sisters before leaving for the hospital. Siblings need to have a chance to ask questions and to cry if they need to.

When hospitalizations are a repeated experience the other children, if old enough, should accompany the family to be present during the entire process. Children over 5 or 6 can help amuse a hospitalized brother or sister, and can benefit from sharing a difficult experience with the family. Otherwise, they may not understand the tension of the parents and may resent the attention and new toys the hospitalized brother or sister gets. It will not hurt children to comfort a mother who cries as her child goes to surgery. On the contrary, if children can share in the family's pain they will be better able to share in the family's joys.

THE PARENTS' OWN NEEDS

During the infancy and early years of a child with a disability, the parents have a massive task in getting to know and appreciate the child and her strengths, learning about the disability and the care she needs, and dealing with their own reactions to the event. They may find they have little time and less inclination to pay attention to their own needs as individual people. Their own guilt may interfere. "How can I think of having fun," they say, "when my child has this terrible problem?"

Yet it is not selfish to pay attention to oneself, if only because one can be a better parent, with more to give to children, if one has some measure of personal fulfillment in life. (Of course, there are other reasons too, but if a parent feels a great sense of guilt this may be the only one he or she will be able to respond to at first.) Most parents find that they do not make good martyrs in the long run.

Parents need to make some provisions for growth, relaxation, and fun in their own lives. There are as many ways of doing this as there are personalities in people who become parents of children with disabilities. During very stressful times, a parent's well-being might require asking a friend to babysit while a much-needed nap is taken. Or, the need may be for an understanding person to talk to about the pain. At other times, the need may be for a career or hobbies that are stimulating and enjoyable.

The quality of the marital relationship needs to be attended to too. It is easy for any new parents to become so engrossed in their roles as "parents" that they overlook being lovers and companions to their spouses. This is an especially dangerous trap for parents of a child with a disability. Most people, however, get married in the first place because they enjoy each other and they want to be together, and not just because they want to be parents.

Private times together — to talk, to go for walks or go out to eat, or for sex — may need to be planned for. Many people think that sharing, especially in sex, should not have to be planned for, that it should happen spontaneously. Planning, however, need not detract from the quality of intimacy. Indeed, in the busy lives of most households, it is essential if child care, job concerns, and household maintenance are not to interfere with times for parents to be together. The planning itself can be a contributor to an atmosphere of warmth and sharing. Simply saying, "I want to set aside some time to be alone with you" to a spouse can in itself be a powerful message of love and caring. Partners in a marriage that is to continue to grow and be satisfying to both people need to share more than work, worry, and sorrow. They need to share in lighthearted and tender moments.

QUESTIONS FOR PARENTS

1. How are my child's needs like those of any child of her age or stage of development?
2. How are they different?
3. What things are "normal" children of her age or stage of development doing?
4. How can I best or most easily approximate those experiences?
5. How can I balance the needs of my other children?
6. Do I allow my other children to share in the bad, as well as the good, experiences that we have?
7. Am I remembering to pay attention to my own needs?
8. Am I allowing myself sufficient rest, relaxation, and time away from my child?
9. Do I allow myself to ask for and receive help when I need it?
10. Are my spouse and I allowing enough time for talking, sharing, and deepening our relationship?

REFERENCES

1. Klaus, Marshall H. and Kennell, John H., *Maternal-Infant Bonding*, C.V. Mosby, 1976.
2. Doyle, Phyllis B., Goodman, John F., Grotsky, Jeffrey N. and Mann, Lester, *Helping the Severely Handicapped Child: A Guide for Parents*, Thomas Y. Crowell, 1979.
3. Finnie, Nancie, *Handling the Young Cerebral Palsied Child at Home*, E. P. Dutton, 1975.
4. Brown, Sara L. and Moersch, Martha S., Eds., *Parents on the Team*, University of Michigan Press, 1978.

6

ISSUES OF EARLY CHILDHOOD
The Years From 2 to 5

The effects of a disability are often not readily apparent during infancy. Babies are not expected to be able to talk, walk, use their limbs in a coordinated manner, or be toilet-trained. To some extent, parents' needs to fantasize that there has been a mistake in the diagnosis or even to deny that the disability exists can be allowed to operate. As the child leaves babyhood, however, the disability becomes more obvious. It assumes more reality to the parents. Fantasies and denials no longer serve as well.

The milestones of child development — the usual times for standing, walking, and speech — each can present new evidence of the child's problems. "It takes courage," says Jack Bavin, "to be able to face up to the gradual unveiling of the true picture."[1] As the child learns and progresses in some areas, the deficits or lags in other areas are more obvious. As she begins to outgrow the usual infant seats and strollers and becomes bigger and heavier, questions and issues around the mechanics of daily living loom larger.

The toddler and preschool years are a time when much learning ordinarily takes place. The "average" young child becomes more vigorous in her exploration of the world. She is active and on the go, and needs constant supervision to protect her from accidents. The toddler is also beginning to develop a sense of herself as a person separate from the parents. Her own wishes come in conflict with the wishes of others. She learns that she can say "*no*," and usually does so often enough to frustrate the parents. Her hands are usually busy exploring, manipulating, building, and taking apart.

Some familiarity with this developmental stage will be helpful to parents as they consider how the child's particular disability affects her experiences and learning. They will be better able to plan for providing these natural experiences. The more the child's life can approximate, within her abilities, what it would be if she did not have a disability, the less she is apt to fall farther behind in her developmental progress.

There is, however, a risk involved in using developmental knowledge of nonhandicapped children in thinking about and planning for children with disabilities. The risk is that these "normal" developmental stages and needs may simply not apply to a child with a disability. This child's experience of herself and of the world may be totally different. Her patterns and sequences of learning may follow a logic of their own which is every bit as natural and correct as those we consider to be "normal."

> We cannot take for granted "that theories constructed for able-bodied children can correctly interpret the developmental significance of the handicapped child . . . handicapped children often live in a social world that is radically different from the one inhabited by their able-bodied peers, and their physical or mental disabilities often impose sharp constraints on the ways that they can obtain and analyze experience."[2]

If the handicapped child's world and learning are so different, why consider "normal" developmental stages at all? First, because we have little else to go on. We simply do not know enough about how children with disabilities perceive and process information. Second, many parents become so engrossed in their child's differences and care that they neglect or overlook activities and opportunities that the child could utilize to learn and grow. Parents may continue to do things "for" a child, for example, long after he or she is capable of learning to do them alone.

Information about what is usual for a nonhandicapped child at a given stage of development should be considered, but only as the roughest of starting points. Parents and professionals alike need to be ready to discard preconceived ideas as they learn more about how a particular child reacts to and learns from the world.

LEARNING

The typical toddler likes to balance her daring in explorations with frequent checks on the parents, her source of security. As Verda Heisler puts it, there is a natural alternation of independent self-assertion and dependency. The child can be observed to run bravely forth to play but will run back periodically for hugs from the mother.[3] The ability to do this can be severely restricted for the child with mobility problems, leaving her more vulnerable to conflicts between these opposing forces. The parents of a severely disabled child may not be able to overcome this completely, but any device parental ingenuity can come up with to allow the child some measure of independent movement and play out of the immediate presence of the parent will be useful.

The child of this age is mastering many new skills in speech, control of the body, and use of the hands. Parents of children with disabilities can use play time with their children as opportunities to teach. Parents may want to work closely with their children's physical, occupational, or speech therapist to explore ways of incorporating useful activities into games that can be fun for both child and parent. But not all "play" should be work. The essence of play is pleasure, for both parent and child, and there need to be times that each can simply enjoy the other without worrying about whether the child is learning anything.

Some basic guidelines for teaching children are helpful when the parent does decide that he wishes to do this. These are outlined and discussed more fully by Jack Bavin in Nancie Finnie's *Handling the Young Cerebral Palsied Child at Home.*[1]

1. Choose a time when the child is alert, responsive, and keen to cooperate. For example, teaching feeding skills when the child is hungry will take advantage of his own powerful motivation.

2. In attempting to teach something that involves a sequence of motions, the parent's help should be withdrawn near the end of the sequence first, and gradually closer and closer to the beginning. If the desired goal is to have the child use a spoon to transfer food to his mouth, the parent's hand can guide the movement until the spoon is almost in his mouth at first, and then gradually withdraw earlier as he masters the motion.

3. Lessons should be kept short. Both parents and children will be frustrated if teaching sessions go on beyond the point when something can reasonably be expected to be accomplished. The timing needs to be more closely adapted to the child's attention span than to the parent's desires.

4. Contests of will power should be avoided. If the teaching session deteriorates into a battle between parent and child, the parent will usually lose. It is better to end the session and try again later.

5. Parents need to demonstrate clearly to the child what he or she is expected to do. The child will need to see, often many times, how the task is expected to be performed. Careful demonstrations to show the sequence of activities are especially important to children who are deaf. Other children need to hear words describing what is happening, whether or not they are able to speak themselves.

6. The child needs to be encouraged for his or her efforts and praised for successes. Enthusiasm and praise are important motivating factors, and are better in the long run for both parent and child than scolding or punishment for failures.

Parents may have a difficult time in keeping their own frustration with the child's progress and their deep longing to see her overcome her disability from interfering with their ability to be helpful. It is hard to watch a child struggle with something that comes easily to other children. Parents need an opportunity to express their anger, frustration, and sorrow about the child's difficulties somewhere other than in their interactions with the child. This may be with an understanding friend or relative, another parent in a parent group, or with a professional counselor. Parents need to be assured that such feelings are human and natural, and only cause problems if they are bottled up and hidden, only to surface when the parent is trying to be helpful to the child.

Sometimes, if the parent's frustration is too great, or if the parent and child are locked into a battle of wills, the simplest remedy may be to find someone else who can temporarily take over the teaching. The parent may be unwittingly sending conflicting messages to the child. For example, the parent who is trying to teach a child to walk with crutches may fear underneath that the child is not ready for this and that she will fall and hurt herself. The parent may be unaware of the ways in which she is subtly saying to the child, "This is dangerous. I'm afraid you will get hurt." Sometimes an older sibling, a grandparent, or a babysitter can take over some of the teaching. Or a physical or occupational therapist can be consulted about the possibility of conducting sessions with the child which will be free of the emotional undercurrents of the parent-child relationship.

MOBILITY

During these years the child needs to have provided, if at all possible, some means for her to move herself from one place to another within the house. Homemade boards on casters or hand-operated toys available in stores may be useful for the child with some arm movement. Parents should not forget, of course, that the child also needs ample time to have her hands free to develop dexterity.

Outside the house, wagons or other toys may be used to take her on walks and help her to explore the neighborhood. A cart called the "Bugger" which resembles a rickshaw and is attached to a parent's bicycle can be found in bicycle shops. These allow the child to experience faster movement and to share in outings with the rest of the family. Outdoor equipment such as sleds and swings can often be adapted with extra supports and safety belts. Light-weight, collapsible strollers in larger sizes are now on the market and may enable the parent to avoid purchasing a heavier, more expensive wheelchair until later.

Parents who are considering the purchase of special equipment need to become familiar with the range of items available on the market and to think specifically about what they wish to achieve through the use of the item. Diane B. D'Eugenio lists the following points to be considered:[4]

1. Will it meet the child's needs? These needs must be clearly defined and broken down into their components before this question can be answered.
2. How long will it be needed? Can it be adjusted or otherwise altered to last longer?
3. What are the difficulties with it? For example, does it fit into the spaces available; can it be moved easily?
4. What is the cost of the item? Can it be rented or borrowed?

A careful thinking through of what is to be accomplished by using a particular piece of equipment can help to avoid costly mistakes in purchasing. Parents who consult with physical and occupational therapists and other parents in parent groups can often come up with less expensive alternatives. The members of a parents' association will ordinarily have years of experience in modifying and adapting everyday household items to meet their children's needs. Often, parent groups will not only share ideas, instructions and blueprints but will arrange to swap or resell outgrown items. If the child's physician agrees that a piece of equipment is necessary and must be purchased, a written prescription for the item can be used to deduct the cost at tax time.

The child's doctor will decide when and with what kind of mechanical assistance the child should begin standing and walking. Parents will want to be sure that they understand the rationale for and use of the quipment chosen. Specific instructions for helping the child and carrying out any prescribed exercises are necessary. New shoes and braces should be removed frequently during the first few days of use and the skin inspected to be sure that pressure spots do not exist.

Braces, crutches, walkers, and other orthopedic appliances should increase the child's ability to move about in an upright position, or in a manner more like the way that other people move about. The parent who watches the expression of joy on a young child's face as she realizes she can walk about often comes to a startling realization: children do not view their mobility aids as the rest of the world does.

While parents may have been accustomed to thinking of braces and crutches as encumbrances, and children who are using them as "confined" to them, to the child they are exactly the opposite. They represent freedom. Even wheelchairs mean freedom from being restricted to sitting in one spot. Parents who share in their child's joy as she learns to use her equipment must undergo a radical change in their thinking. Things that previously were thought of with sorrow or even pity are now vehicles for freedom. Their use is actually celebrated. This ability to shift dramatically how things are defined is an important element in parents' capacity not only to cope but also to find new sources of joy and satisfaction.

The child during these years is beginning to grow larger and heavier and can no longer be lifted and carried as easily as a baby. It is none too early for parents consciously to develop patterns of safe lifting to protect their own backs and muscles. Proper lifting means keeping the back straight and letting the leg muscles do most of the work. To lift correctly:

1. Get close to the child. You can't let your legs do the work if your arms are outstretched. Have the item you are going to be lifting the child to nearby.
2. Squat, don't bend at the waist. Remember, the back should be straight. Have one foot slightly forward (in the direction you will be going).
3. Get a good grip on the child. As you rise upward, the leg muscles should be doing the work while the back muscles simply hold the back steady.
4. Go as short a distance as possible. If you must change direction, do it by pivoting on your feet, not by twisting the body.
5. If you can slide the child's bottom onto your thigh while you are kneeling, with one hand under her knees and the other around her shoulders, your thigh will be the support for most of her weight as you rise.

Sketches of proper lifting can be found in *Helping the Severely Handicapped Child*,[5] or parents can ask their own physicians for instructions for proper lifting and back care.

As the child grows out of infancy, clothing may become more of a concern for three reasons. One is that the child who is crawling on the floor past the age when children usually begin to walk needs clothing that will protect the sensitive skin of paralyzed legs and yet not be torn to shreds too readily by the rough treatment it receives. A second is that various forms of bracing may be prescribed for the child, necessitating clothing that will fit well either under or over the braces. And the third is that garments may need to be taken on and off as easily as possible so that the child who learns slowly or who has trouble coordinating her movements can begin to take over dressing and undressing herself.

The legs and feet of the child who lacks muscle function and sensation in these limbs must be protected from injury as she moves about. If she is not yet wearing braces and brace shoes, soft shoes can be worn. Socks need to fit correctly with neither bunching nor tight binding at any point. Cotton or cotton blends are preferable to nylon, although synthetic fibers that stretch are less likely to bunch up in the shoes. Outer pants may need to be as sturdy as possible (denim, for example) with the softer cottons reserved for special occasions, especially if the child enjoys crawling outside on concrete. Extra patches for reinforcement can be ironed or sewn in over spots that receive the most wear and tear. Overall-style pants work best for the child who tends to lose his slacks as he pulls himself along the floor. Girls can wear smock-type blouses that do not get caught under their knees as longer dresses do. Limbs that lack sensation are also more vulnerable to the effects of cold weather and frostbite. Extra layers underneath snowpants or a sleeping bag zipped over the legs may be used for additional protection from the cold.

As the child who still wears diapers gets too large for the toddler size pants with snaps along the inside seams of the legs, parents may wish to alter slacks to include Velcro strip closures along these seams for ease in toileting or changing. Velcro strips in clothing are useful for many people, whether for the convenience of the parent or for the child who is learning to dress herself. Parents should remember to be sure that the strips are closed before placing them in the washing machine or they will snag other clothing.

It is easy for the parent to continue to dress the child with a disability long after she should be learning to do it on her own. Households are often busy and rushed in the morning, and certainly the parent can do the job with more efficiency and less frustration than the child. But this is not the way for the child to learn independence.

If the job of dressing herself completely seems to be too much for the child to tackle all at once, the parent can proceed in stages. For instance, the parent can do all of the dressing except for one item (the shirt or the slacks) and leave the child with that while the parent packs the lunches or brushes her teeth. If the child is retarded, the task of putting on one item of clothing may need to be broken down further into each component movement, and the child given an opportunity to practice each one separately.

Clothing should be as simple as possible for the child who has difficulty in controlling his movements or in fine hand coordination. Buttons should be large, rather than small; loops can be attached to the ends of zippers to make them easier to pull; and Velcro can be used instead of buttons or snaps for closures. Parents may wish to write to the National Easter Seal Society for Crippled Children and Adults for a copy of *Self-Help Clothing for Handicapped Children* by Clari Bare, Eleanor Boettke, and Neva Waggoner. The address is: 2023 West Ogden Avenue, Chicago, Illinois 60612.

BOWEL AND BLADDER MANAGEMENT

As the child approaches 3 years of age, issues of bowel and bladder management or training are likely to be of concern to parents. It is the age at which parents can usually expect gradually to withdraw from the responsibility of diapering and toileting their children. Both physical and mental disabilities can make it impossible for these expectations to be met at this time. Thus this becomes yet another reminder for parents of the reality of the disability. Parents can experience underlying anger that the level of care needed is "more than they bargained for."

It may help for parents to remember that there is a wider variation in the "normal" ages for achievement of bowel and bladder control than we often think. Many children without disabilities do not achieve full control until closer to 5 years of age. We hope that the days when early toilet training was seen as a measure of parental success and competence are over. Because there are differences of approach to children who have problems with bowel and bladder control because the nerve supply to these areas has been damaged and children who take longer to learn voluntary control because they are retarded, these areas will be discussed separately.

Children with Physical Disabilities

Any condition that affects the spinal cord can also affect the nerves that control bladder and bowel functions. Children with spina bifida, for example, usually have some involvement of these nerves in spite of wide variations in the degree of paralysis in their feet, legs, and hips. While the child with nerve damage will not be "trained" in the sense that she will have the kind of voluntary control over the muscles that empty the bowel and bladder that other children might, successful management programs are possible.

Urinary management in the child who lacks a functioning nerve supply to the bladder has two main objectives: preservation of the health of his kidneys, and achievement of a method of collecting urine that allows her as much independence and freedom from social embarrassment as possible.

The child whose bladder functions have been affected by the disability needs to be evaluated early and regularly by a urologist. The first evaluation should take place in the first few months of life and after that at least yearly unless the urologist recommends more frequent checkups. Infection or inadequate drainage of urine can lead to potentially life-threatening kidney damage. This may occur without the child showing any outward signs of sickness. Yearly x-rays of the urinary tract (called intravenous pyelograms, or IVPs) and periodic testing of the urine for bacteria (urine cultures) can provide the reassurance that the child's kidneys are remaining healthy. Sometimes minor but persistent signs such as listlessness or loss of appetite can alert the parent to request a urine culture to be sure that infection is not the cause. Other tests of bladder functioning may be necessary from time to time to safeguard health and to help determine the most realistic management program.

Once the safety of the urinary tract is taken care of, the next question is: how shall the elimination of urine be handled so that the child can stay dry for reasonable periods of time and not be embarrassed? There are no uniform answers to this question for there are individual variations in how much a child's bladder will expand to hold urine and whether it empties completely or not. It used to be that the awful choice for parents was between diapers and major surgery to bypass the bladder so that the urine drains into a pouch worn on the abdomen. Fortunately, this is no longer the case. Other alternatives are available and more can be anticipated as research into these areas continues. Parents will need to consult a urologist who is experienced in dealing with children with a lack of nerve supply to the bladder and who is sensitive to the needs of children to deal with this as independently as "normally" as possible.

The most popular alternative at this time is intermittent self-catheterization. This involves the insertion of a small tube, or catheter, into the urinary opening at regular intervals to drain the bladder. Children are usually taught to do this themselves, although parents may initially perform this for the very young child. Sometimes, medications are also used which act to influence the ability of the bladder to expand or to release urine. Straining or the application of external pressure over the bladder (the Crede maneuver) may also be used. None of these are "self-help" solutions; a urologist's help in determining which programs should be attempted is crucial, because some of the very "simple" solutions can be dangerous to some children. For example, the application of pressure over the bladder area can force urine back up towards the kidneys in a reverse direction if the tendency for this (called reflux) is present in a particular child.

Some children wear sanitary napkins or "minipads" to deal with occasional leaking. While large-size diapers are available from some specialized sources, other alternatives are far preferable for the child who, like most, finds this humiliating. Boys may be able to use an external collecting device which fits over the penis like a condom. External devices are less satisfactory in girls.

One surgical approach to the problem of incontinence in some children with impaired bladder function is the implantation of an artificial sphincter. This relatively new approach involves a silicone rubber cuff which, when inflated, serves to close off the flow of urine through the urethra. When it is deflated by squeezing a small pumping device in the scrotum or in the labia, it allows urine to flow through.

Sometimes, surgery to enlarge the urinary openings may be useful in promoting drainage. The more major procedures of disconnecting the ureters (the tubes which lead from each kidney to the bladder) from the bladder and allowing them to drain through an opening into a pouch worn on the abdomen, are rarely used today for achieving social acceptance. They may be useful however if all other methods have failed or if the kidneys are in danger. Parents whose children have had this surgery or who are contemplating it may wish to contact the United Ostomy Association, 2001 W. Beverly Blvd., Los Angeles, California 90057.

Lack of bowel control is, fortunately, not as great a problem for the child's health as is urinary incontinence. For the parent, and for the child as she grows older, however, regular evacuation of stool with a minimal incidence of accidents becomes extremely important. While the child will not be "toilet-trained" in the same sense as a child with normal nerve supply to the bowel, she should be able to move gradually toward a predictable and manageable schedule.

Generally, the establishment of a regular bowel schedule involves two components: diet and timing. The child's diet will need to be regulated so that the stools are neither too soft nor hard, small lumps. Parents should be aware that small amounts of loose, watery stools may actually represent overflow around severe constipation and may require medical advice. Attention to the diet usually does not involve tedious or meticulous meal planning. Once a parent discovers which foods (usually only a few) are apt to cause loose or runny stools, these are simply avoided. The diet should be generally well-balanced and contain sufficient roughage, fruits, vegetables, and fluids. Sources of roughage in addition to fruits and vegetables are brans, some berries, nuts, and smaller amounts of sugar and refined flours. Parents can consult with the child's doctor or a dietician if they are having difficulty in achieving consistency of the stools. For constipation, Karo syrup, prune juice, or commercial stool softeners may be useful.

From the age of 2 or 3, the child should be placed on a comfortable potty chair at the time of day when she has been observed to be likely to have a bowel movement. Her feet should be on the floor, and her torso should be comfortably supported so that she has no fear of falling. If the child can contract the abdominal muscles, she can do this to help initiate bowel action. Or she may lean forward with her abdomen on her thighs or blow up a balloon to achieve a similar effect.

The establishment of a regular time each day for evacuation is important. Parents will need patience; it may take some time and experimentation to achieve a predictable schedule. For many children, 20 to 30 minutes after breakfast is the optimal time. This timing takes advantage of the body's natural gastrocolic reflex, in which the taking in of food stimulates activity in other parts of the intestinal tract.

Various methods for stimulating the bowel may be useful while the schedule is being established. When the pattern is firmly established, these can often be dropped. These methods may include suppositories or Fleet enemas. Suppositories can be inserted 15 to 30 minutes before the anticipated bowel movement. If needed, nonallergenic tape can be used to hold the buttocks together. A finger protected with a disposable finger cot can be used to provide gental manual stimulation of the rectum. Manual removal of stool, however, is not recommended because of the risk of injury to the surface of the bowel.

Children who are Retarded

The mastery of control of bladder and bowel elimination will of course take longer in the child who is retarded. Again, parents should keep in mind that some children without disabilities do not achieve full control until close to 5 years of age. Parents will need to assess the child's readiness to begin training in order to spare both themselves and the child frustration caused by beginning too early. Positive answers to the following questions indicate that training might be feasible:

1. Does the child show, in other areas, a desire to be in control or to please others?
2. Does he or she show signs of discomfort when wet or soiled, or otherwise show some understanding of the difference between wet and dry?
3. Does he or she show some bodily clues or signs that indicate elimination is about to occur?
4. Can the child participate in some of the necessary activities such as pulling pants up and down, or washing hands?
5. Is the child willing to sit on the potty chair?
6. Is the relationship between parent and child reciprocal and helpful?
7. Does the parent have the time to be consistent and encouraging during the training?

When the parent has decided that attempting training is feasible, he or she will need to discover the patterns in the child's elimination. Keeping a record for a week or two of the child's intake of food and fluids and the times of bowel movements and urination can help to clarify useful patterns. The parent will also probably want to decide on a reward to use for the child when she is successful or when she has made efforts to cooperate. This may be a small amount of her favorite cereal, words of praise, or a hug. The child should be healthy and eating an adequate diet.

The tasks involved in independent toileting need to be identified and broken down into small, specific behaviors. Each phase — removing clothing, sitting on the toilet or potty seat, eliminating, wiping, replacing clothing, and washing and drying hands — has many individual components that may have to be worked on separately.

Parents need to remember that learning these behaviors and activities takes longer for the child who is retarded. Each improvement, no matter how small, should be recognized and rewarded. The most difficult part for parents is probably continuing to ignore the accidents or mistakes while praising the efforts and successes. But the child needs positive reinforcement of her success with each individual part of the sequence, even if she has made a mistake in another part. If the child has an accident, the clothing should be changed as soon as possible so that she does not get used to being wet. She can be shown "wetness" by touching the wet pants and helping to change herself, but she should not be scolded or punished.

Bowel and bladder taining are reasonable goals for most children who are retarded even though the motor activity and physical and social awareness the child needs are quite complex. The learning process does take longer. If parents are becoming frustrated with slow results, they may wish to rethink the sequence of behaviors to see if they can be broken down even further. Perhaps the activities are still too complicated and need to be in even simpler steps. Or, they may wish to discontinue training temporarily until the child seems more ready or the parent feels more optimistic and capable of patience.

ESTABLISHING LIMITS FOR THE CHILD

The young child learns about the world and herself not only by her explorations but also by the limits defined for her by the adults in her world. Slowly, she learns from the people who care for her that some activities earn disapproval or pain. She learns that sometimes she must wait for a wish to be granted: that cookies come after lunch, or that Mommy will not take her out in the snow until she has finished her chores. She realizes that while her brother may get to lick the extra frosting off of the beaters today, the next time a cake is baked it will be her turn for this treat.

Often parents teach these lessons to "normal" children naturally and easily, without even being aware that they are imparting important lessons about getting along in the world. But this may be very much more difficult when the child has a disability. Suddenly, each limit, each "deprivation", that parents would ordinarily impose on another child without much thought becomes loaded with other meanings and implications.

Parents may wish to "make up" to this child for all the other deprivations in her life, or for the pain and fear she experienced in the hospital last week. Hidden guilt about the things parents can do that she cannot makes the parents wish to spare her any further pain or frustration. On the other hand, parents can usually see perfectly clearly that the child has all the makings of a perfect tyrant who will loudly and vociferously demand that her wishes be granted immediately. Parents are at war within themselves, and each time they must decide whether Susie or her brothers get to lick the bowl today they try to do so without acknowledging the meanings of these things for them. It is no wonder that such everyday decisions are so difficult.

As parents try to deal matter-of-factly with these never-ending minor decisions of life, they cannot understand why they seem so difficult or why they seem to arouse such a confused welter of feelings. They cannot explain why they sometimes wish to pamper and indulge the child, while at other times they are filled with the urge to scream at her.

Children *do* need limits, and from a very early age. They need the security of knowing that parents will stop them before they get out of control or do something dangerous. They also need to begin to learn to accomodate to the other people in the world who have their own rights, wishes, and possessions. Parents who have difficulty in setting limits or in sticking to them may want to think about the following suggestions.

1. Keep firmly in mind what kind of person you hope your child will be and how you would like other people to react to him or her. Most parents do not wish to raise a spoiled child who has little consideration for other people. Having a firm base on which to make decisions will enable parents to remain calmer and make more consistent judgments.

2. Be sure to praise or reward behaviors that are desirable. The child needs to be encouraged for what he or she does right as well as corrected for what he or she does wrong.

3. Recognize how your own feelings of guilt or anger enter into the difficulty in setting limits for the child. Don't deny the feelings,

but find another place to work on them. This can be with a friend, a clergyman, or a professional counselor.

4. Attend meetings of groups of parents of children with disabilities. There you will meet other parents who struggle with the same conflicts. You can get the relief of knowing you are not alone, bizarre, or evil, as well as learning concrete and practical suggestions for dealing with everyday situations.

There are, of course, vast differences in children with respect to how much "trouble" they get into. Some children are very passive by nature; parents of children like this may find themselves almost looking for things to correct the child for. At the other extreme are children who seem to need little sleep and who are constantly on the go. Parents of these children may need to pay more attention to their own needs for rest and relaxation so that they can better cope when they are caring for their children.

Issues and behaviors that are upsetting to parents, such as a child's refusal to eat certain foods or use the toilet, are the most likely places to become battlegrounds between parents and young children. While no parent should expect to be perfectly calm and consistent in dealings with young children, it is certainly easier to maintain a reasonable degree of equanimity if the parent has had sufficient rest and opportunities for "time off." Often, a parent also needs a wider perspective. If Johnny does not eat vegetables for certain days or even weeks, this will not cause any difficulties if he eats other nourishing food, is in reasonably good health, and has a reasonably balanced diet over a period of months. The diet does not have to be perfectly balanced each day.

Many young children will resort to tantrums when they are tired or frustrated. If the tantrums do not succeed in getting the child what he wants, they are likely to be used only sporadically and will disappear relatively quickly. Parents must steel themselves to ignore tantrum behavior firmly to be sure that the child does not learn that such behaviors "work." This can be very difficult if the tantrum occurs in public.

At the same time, it may be worthwhile to take a look at the child's overall situation. Does the child get enough positive attention and stimulation? Have there been any recent disruptions in the household or the routines that may be upsetting, especially to the child who is retarded? Sometimes, an abrupt change in parental demands can confuse a child and trigger the onset of tantrums.[1] Parents may want to consider whether they have recently begun to expect more from the child for any reason.

Head banging, rocking, and other forms of repetitive body movements may be disturbing behaviors to families and may be difficult to eliminate once they are established. These too may be signals that the child needs more stimulation. Many kinds of disturbing behaviors in children may be attempts to get attention, even though the attention they produce is often negative. For example, a child who cannot speak or run about may scream when she is bored, frustrated, or angry. If she learns that when she screams, an adult will rush to give comfort and attention, she will continue to use this behavior.

Parents and babysitters can pay more attention to the more subtle aspects of the child's responses, her eyes, or her voice, so that she will not need to yell louder to get attention. To eliminate the undesirable behaviors, the necessary attention and stimulation — hugs, play, conversation and toys — need to be provided when the child is not using the behaviors. When the behaviors serve no useful purpose for the child they will usually fade away.

PRESCHOOL EXPERIENCES

As the child with the disability reaches the age of 2 or 2½, it is time to begin to think about experiences for the child outside the home. Many families may not have made use of nursery schools or preschools for their other children, and may wonder why this should be considered for the child with a disability. Other children in the family may not have started school until kindergarten, and may have done very well. Some parents may have strong underlying wishes to protect their child from the hurts of the world. They may wish to keep her surrounded by love in his own home for as long as possible. These wishes may be normal and natural. But sometimes, they are fed by underlying guilt and the need of the parent to "make up" to the child for the condition that she has.

The child with a disability, even if she has brothers and sisters in the home, can benefit from the opportunity to play and interact on a regular basis with other children of her own age. She is bound to miss out on some of the activities and experiences that nondisabled children have during these years. Preschool experiences, with opportunities for additional learning and social experiences, can help to compensate for these lacks so that she will be better prepared for grade school.

Many children with disabilities are familiar with two environments: home and hospital. A good preschool can provide an extra dimension to the child's life with a warm and stimulating environment. In addition, it can offer play and learning materials and activities that are not convenient or practical to have at home. Sand tables and complete childsize kitchens are not feasible in most households but are commonplace in nursery schools. A good preschool program can also help to identify special learning needs that the child may have and provide learning experiences to meet those needs.

Some parents will welcome the opportunity for the child to learn and be cared for elsewhere for a few hours a day. They will use these hours to restore and enrich themselves, or to work at necessary household tasks or jobs outside the home. Others will feel guilty about sending the child "away." For many families, a real danger exists that the family, and the parents in particular, will make the child and her needs the center of their lives, submerging their own interests and needs. Nursery school experience can help provide parents with another viewpoint of the child and her capabilities. This is helpful in reinforcing the separateness of parent and child.

It is now national policy to begin the education of children with handicaps by at least 3 years of age. The Education of All Handicapped Children Act (PL 94-142) authorizes and encourages states to provide these programs with incentive grants. Some states provide for the education of children with disabilities between ages 3 to 5 and 18 to 21, while others still do not. Parents can call their local school districts for information about public preschool programs in their area.

Head Start programs provide diagnostic, educational, health, nutritional, and other services to preschool children who are educationally disadvantaged. The Head Start authorization states that 10 percent of spaces shall be reserved for children who have handicaps.

Parents who want to explore the full range of preschool programs will want to contact voluntary agencies in their area (Associations for the Retarded, United Cerebral Palsy, etc.) for information on existing preschool programs. They may also wish to contact private nursery and preschools if the cost of these is feasible for the family. Just because a preschool program has never had a child with a disability enrolled in it, does not necessarily mean that a particular child could not do very well there and benefit other children as well as herself. Early childhood is a perfect time to begin a child's attendance in classes of children who do not have disabilities. Young children typically show a brief spurt of open curiosity about things like wheelchairs, crutches, or speech problems. If their questions are briefly and honestly answered, they will proceed readily to accept the child with a disability into their activities. Parents will want to visit programs, observe sessions, and talk with teachers about the program and their own child's needs before making a decision.

QUESTIONS FOR PARENTS

1. Do I have an understanding of what my child's developmental needs are at his or her age and stage of development?
2. Does my child have ample opportunities for stimulation and different play materials?
3. If my child has mobility problems, can I find, or improvise, a way for him or her to experience movement?
4. Do I have a sense of my child's development as a separate person with his or her own individuality?
5. Are my own needs, and those of others in my family, being met?
6. Do I have someone with whom I can talk over the frustrations of daily life?
7. Can I correct my child's behavior and set limits for him or her without feeling upset or guilty?
8. Am I familiar with preschool programs in my area? What are the advantages and disadvantages of each for my child and our family?

REFERENCES

1. Bavin, Jack, In Finnie, Nancie, Ed., *Handling the Young Cerebral Palsied Child at Home*, E. P. Dutton, 1975.
2. Gliedman, John and Roth, William, *The Unexpected Minority: Handicapped Children in America*, For the Carnegie Council on Children, Harcourt, Brace, Jovanovich, 1980.
3. Heisler, Verda, *A Handicapped Child in the Family: A Guide for Parents*, Grune and Stratton, 1972.
4. D'Eugenio, Diane B., In Brown, Sara L., and Moersch, Martha S., Eds., *Parents on the Team*, University of Michigan Press, 1978.
5. Doyle, Phyllis B., Goodman, John F., Grotsky, Jeffrey N. and Mann, Lester, *Helping the Severely Handicapped Child: A Guide for Parents and Teachers*, Thomas Y. Crowell, 1979.

7
WHAT SORT OF EDUCATION?

As the child with a disability approaches school age, new and complex issues arise for parents. Some of these relate to the feelings and concerns aroused in the parent who must contemplate sending the child out of the home and into the "real world." Others have to do with the need to gain some understanding of the complexities of the learning needs of the child, his educational rights under the law, and the differences in educational philosophies and programs. Again, parents are called upon to make decisions in areas that are usually outside the realm of their experience and expertise, decisions that may have a profound impact on the child's life and development.

The first day of school is often a momentous occasion in the life of any child. Parents experience many emotions as they watch a child go off on the school bus for the first time: pride, anticipation, worry, and sadness that a phase of the child's life in the family has ended. These may be accentuated when the child has a disability. For many children with disabilities, the beginning of school may be the first real confrontation with the outside world and its expectations. Parents are forced to view the child not only from their own perspective but with the added dimension of how they imagine he is seen through the eyes of others.

The field of education for children with disabilities has undergone a radical change in recent years. It is easy, in our confusion about what is optimal for each child, to lose sight of just how new this major change is. Until the mid-1970s, the prevailing philosophy was: if a child did not "fit" into the public school system, his education was the parent's responsibility. Local school districts were not held responsible for educating all children with handicaps. The change came about because of a growing awareness of the unfairness of offering the right of a "free, public education" to some children and not to others. This awareness did not come about entirely spontaneously. It was created, in large part, by the concerted efforts of parents' organizations and civil liberties groups.

The Education for All Handicapped Children Act (Public Law 94-142) passed in November, 1975, is the landmark exemplifying the new philosophy. There are three major concepts embodied in PL 94-142, which provides for a free, appropriate public education in the least restrictive environment. The first is that every child, regardless of disability, is entitled to a free, public education. The responsibility is thus placed squarely with the school district. The second major concept is that this education must be *appropriate* to the child's needs. No longer must the child "fit" into standard programs to qualify. And third, this education must be provided in the *least restrictive* environment. Automatic segregation of children with disabilities is no longer acceptable.

The passage of Public Law 94-142 was viewed as a major victory by parents and others concerned about educational opportunities for children with handicaps. At long last, the educational rights of these children seemed to be spelled out in the law. Parents were relieved that they could at last stand on solid legal ground in their negotiations with local school districts.

But our society has still not adequately faced the question of where the financial responsibility for this education belongs. Public Law 94-142 is meaningless without the funds to do the job, and the question of whether there will be adequate funding remains in grave doubt. The struggles to improve the nation's economic situation have led to proposals with the potential to undercut the support necessary for implementation of the concepts of P.L. 94-142. Proposals for distribution for "block grants" to be distributed to states mean a return to the days when state and local governments can decide whether or in what manner they choose to fund education for handicapped children.

There are already extreme variations throughout the country in the amount of money spent per pupil in special education services. According to Brewer and Kakalik, "A child's receipt of special education assistance, and the amount he receives, are unmistakably and strongly dependent on where his parents live."[1] These authors also report that one out of every ten families they surveyed had to move to obtain special education. Many gaps still exist. Some children are still not receiving needed services, while others are receiving services that are inadequate or less than correct. Local school districts are faced simultaneously with increased demands and severe budgetary pressures.

This situation is likely to become worse without strong federal support for free appropriate public education in the least restrictive environment. Parents and advocates may once again find themselves engaged in separate, individual negotiations with local school districts. They may be pitted in these struggles against their own friends and neighbors who hold different expectations for the use of block grants. The lesson to be learned from all of this is that, apparently, the issues of education for those with disabilities will not be resolved until the basic questions of who is responsible and for what are addressed and resolved.

While the conflicts and controversies in our society continue, other more personal issues must be dealt with by families. On an individual family level, the basic dilemma is often: What *is* "appropriate" for this child? Parents may be confused by the professional jargon and diagnostic terms applied to the child and by the variety of educational alternatives. They may be torn by the question of whether it is better for the child to compete in a regular classroom or be more protected in a special classroom.

Real conflicts of opinion do exist as to what is best for a particular child. For example, there is a genuine diversity of opinion as to whether it is better for a young child who is deaf to be taught sign language or oral speech for communication. Difficult situations arise when different "experts" make different recommendations for a child or when the parent does not agree with the recommendations.

Disagreements may center around three major areas. First, parents and school personnel may disagree on the basic question of whether or not the child is "exceptional" and in need of special education. Not all children with disabilities need special education services. These may be termed disagreements of evaluation. Second, there may be differences of opinion as to *what* handicap the child does have, or disagreements of classification. Many disabilities do not present themselves as clearly defined entities. Some parents find that they must continue for years without an accurate diagnosis of their child's problem. And third, there may be disagreements about placement, as to what program is most appropriate for the child.

In the light of such complexities, what are parents to base their decisions on? Parents, of course, cannot see into the future any better than anyone else. Decisions must be made, but parents cannot know in advance that their child will be happy or do well in a particular program. Parents can, however, remember that decisions can be reviewed and altered if experience shows that they are not working well for the child. A parental decision need not be a life sentence. Parents can make their decisions by thinking through the following three areas.

1. The parent's own knowledge of the child. Parents have lived intimately with the child for years, and have had ample opportunity to observe the child's strengths and weaknesses, and how he learns best. They have had to teach the child many things at home and have learned by trial and error some of the approaches that work and some that don't. Parents need to use this knowledge and their own intuitive sense about the child. A program being considered for the child should seem logical — it should "make sense" — in light of what the parent already knows about the child.

2. Professional recommendations and test results. These are important pieces of information to weigh when making educational decisions for the child. Parents need to obtain the recommendations of professionals they trust, and to seek another opinion if there seems to be doubt about the nature of the child's needs. Many kinds of tests can be administered to children. These can provide useful information if it is remembered that all tests have limitations and are best used as indicators or guides, not as infallible "gospel."

3. The child's rights, and the rights of parents, under the law. Parents need to understand clearly what children are entitled to and how they can proceed if they find that they disagree with the recommendations of school officials. This may seem to be a great deal to learn, but the parent does not have to begin from scratch. Much of the collecting of information has already been done (see Appendix B, Education, for listings of publications). Locally, parents can contact parent and disability groups for information and help with problems. They can attend hearings and committee and task force meetings on education issues to learn about their local situation and to meet the people involved in decision-making in their community. There is much help available from other parents and advocates who already "know the ropes."

What does PL 94-142 mean in practical terms to parents of a child with a disability? It means, first and foremost, that every child is entitled to a public education, regardless of his handicap. Beyond this, there are a number of concepts and procedures encompassed in the law of which parents need to have a basic understanding.

THE "LEAST RESTRICTIVE ENVIRONMENT"

The intent of the law is that each child shall receive an education appropriate to his specific needs in the least restrictive environment. Further, the law states that to "the maximum extent appropriate handicapped children will be educated with children who are not handicapped." A careful reading of these words seems to indicate that the intent is primarily to provide the child with the education that he needs, with that education to be provided in the setting that is least restrictive to the child.

"Mainstreaming" is a word that has been applied to this intent, and it is often misunderstood and misused. Mainstreaming is sometimes interpreted as indiscriminately returning all children with special needs to regular classrooms. As Betty Pendler says, "Sometimes the definition means nothing constructive in the educational services — merely a removal of a label and a return to a regular class."[2] Mainstreaming is not "dumping." This is a prospect that strikes fear in the hearts of parents and public school teachers alike.

Application of the intent of mainstreaming means that there should be a range of special assistance available to choose from. A child could be placed in a regular classroom; he could be in a regular class with specific assistance or support services in certain areas; he could be based in a regular class but go to a special classroom or resource room for certain subjects; he could be in a special classroom in a regular school with nonacademic experiences shared with "regular" students; or he could be in a specialized program. Equal opportunity under the law does not necessarily mean equal placement in identical programs. The Council for Exceptional Children defines equal opportunity as "equal access to differing resources for differing objectives." In other words, each child should have an equal chance to have his educational needs met, although the means chosen to meet those needs will not be the same for all children.

In the past, parents were assured by the "experts" in special education that children's needs could best be met in separate programs. The thrust of mainstreaming thus represents a totally different approach and may create anxiety in parents who fear that their children will be rejected by their classmates or will experience failure as they struggle to compete. These worries are real, and need to be addressed openly and honestly. But parents also need to extend their thinking to include not only what the child's needs are now but also what they hope for his future. What kind of a life does the parent foresee for the child? These are painful issues to consider. But if the parent wishes that the child as an adult will be able to live and move about in the world, even if he needs some assistance to do so, the rationale for allowing the child to learn about the nonhandicapped world in childhood becomes clearer.

Parents may have conflicting feelings about mainstreaming, and if they read about the issues involved they will find that educators, too, vary in their feelings and opinions. The debate is further obscured by the fact that the philosophical bases for the discussions are not clear. How we ask the questions about mainstreaming makes a critical difference. Do we ask, "Is the child ready?" or, "Is the school ready?"

Charles Lusthaus and Evelyn Lusthaus write, "By asking when a child is ready for mainstreaming, we are putting the 'burden of proof' on the child. This question has an implicit assumption that the handicapped child is the one who has the responsibility of getting ready — that he must meet some standard in order to fit into the 'mainstream'." Instead, they suggest, the question ought to be, "Is the educational system ready to meet the needs of my child in the least restrictive setting, regardless of his handicaps or disabilities? If not, why is it not ready? What must be done to make it ready?"[3]

Burton Blatt, writing in the same issue of *The Exceptional Parent*, states it even more forcefully. "Not only should mainstreaming be the 'treatment of choice' . . . it should be the assumed treatment unless specifically indicated otherwise . . . The major burden of proof is on the school and the parent to demonstrate that the integrated program is *not* preferable."[4]

Parents may find, in discussing their child's placement with school personnel, that some of the people feel that the child is "not ready." Rather than launching immediately into a major philosophical argument, parents should first ask for more information on the specific reason that the person feels the child is not ready. Is it the child's ability? His learning needs? His behaviors? His frustration tolerance? When the parents learns why the school person feels as he does, the parent is in a better position to state his own case. The parent may not feel that the reasons given are adequate contraindications for a regular school placement. Or the parent may feel that a problem-solving approach can result in the "difficulty" being worked out satisfactorily.

Any placement for a child with special learning needs, if it is to be successful, requires careful consideration of how those needs are to be met. This thought and planning is essential whether the placement is to be in a regular classroom, a special classroom, or a combination of both. Obviously, parents do not want their children subjected to hostile or fearful classmates and teachers. Parents who try to establish a relationship of cooperative partnership with the child's teachers will have a better basis for dealing with problems when and if they do arise.

How can this partnership between parent and teacher be established? Parents need to meet with the child's teachers and indicate their willingness to share information and resolve problems. Some of the areas parents may want to consider are the following.

1. The parent can begin by assuming that the teacher has the child's best interests at heart. Although it may be true that, over the child's school career, the parent may encounter some teachers who do not, at least the parent will know that the problem is not

that he or she didn't give the teacher the benefit of the doubt. Parents are entitled to be treated with respect by the child's teachers; but this obligation works both ways.

2. The parent will want to find out what questions or concerns the teacher has. Parents can provide information on the child's needs and give the teacher literature on the child's disability if this seems appropriate. The teacher may worry that the child will become ill, have a seizure, or hurt himself while in school. Parents can provide reassurance about these fears and also let the teacher know how to handle these situations or how to reach the parents.

Parents can take this opportunity to share with the teacher their own concerns about the classroom situation. For example, parents may be worried about how other children will react to the child or whether friendships will develop. Teachers and parents can discuss together ways of answering the questions of other children and encouraging friendships.

3. The teacher may feel that he or she needs some help in successfully meeting special needs of children in the classroom. Rather than becoming the teacher's adversaries, parents can join *with* the teacher in exploring ways to meet classroom needs. Perhaps the child himself can manage more than the teacher anticipates; or, assistance from resource teachers or teacher aides may be indicated. Parents have options that teachers do not have in prodding the system to be more responsive. Parents have access, through parent organizations and lobbying groups, to sources of pressure on the system that are not available to teachers. The very fact that the parent *wants* to help the teacher find a workable solution can be the best basis for a cooperative relationship.

4. The parent and teacher will need to agree in advance how, and how often, they will communicate about the child's progress. Will communication be by notes sent back and forth with the child? By telephone? By conferences? Getting the ground rules straight at the beginning of the year can avoid unpleasant surprises later on. Parents and teachers need to have a mechanism for communicating problems to each other as they arise.

5. Parents will want to share their concerns with the child's teacher as they come up and before they build up into insurmountable problems. Problems need to be presented as the parent experiences them without attempting to blame anyone. For example, the parent may say, "I am concerned because Susie reports that she's being teased and picked on in school." This kind of statement expresses both the parent's concern and the evidence it is based on, but it also allows the teacher to contribute his or her own perceptions before solutions are considered. The teacher may feel that Susie is being overly sensitive; or that one or two children are indeed insensitive to Susie and can be

talked to individually; or that the problem is more widespread. Choosing an effective approach to the problem requires an accurate definition of what the problem really is.

Such a problem-solving approach will not resolve all difficult situations, but it will allow for the resolution of many potential problems before they become major issues. Occasionally, a parent and teacher will have real difficulties in working together. In such a situation, the parent may want to discuss the matter with someone else who can provide another viewpoint, such as the school principal, or the child's guidance counselor. Parents may wish to request a change of teacher for the child, but they should be certain that it is for the child's benefit, not the parents'.

EVALUATION

P.L. 94-142 provides for children with disabilities, or those who may be potentially in need of special education services, to be tested. This testing may be for two purposes: identification, or to assess whether or not the child does need special education; or evaluation, to determine what the educational needs are and what the placement should be. Parents must be informed by the school of the intent to administer testing or evaluation, and must give their consent, in writing, for these procedures.

The law is quite specific as to what constitutes "evaluation." Evaluation must be done by a multidisciplinary team (often referred to as an "M" team). This team, or group of persons, must include at least one teacher or specialist with knowledge in the area of the suspected disability. The child must be assessed in all areas relating to the suspected disability, including, when appropriate; health, vision, hearing, social and emotional status, general intelligence, academic performance, communicative status, and motor abilities. No single test or group of tests may be used.

When a child is to be assessed through such testing, parents can help prepare him by answering his questions and easing his apprehension. They can also ensure that he comes to the tests after a full night's sleep and a good breakfast. In addition, parents may want to learn more about the purposes of different kinds of tests and their strengths and limitations.

Many different kinds of tests are used in assessing children. Tests may be designed to assess how well a child performs *now*, or to try to predict how well he will do in the future. Parents should understand that tests are only indicators. There is no fixed, permanent "IQ." The same child may score differently on different tests at the same time or on the same test at different times. As Dorothy Dean writes,

"Psychological and intelligence tests are basic diagnostic equipment, but they are like predictions of the weather which may be inaccurate to start with and are susceptible to change. There is no magic in testing that will reveal all that needs to be known about a child's problems and potential."[5] Parents who wish to learn more about tests are referred to *Psychological Testing of Children: A Consumer's Guide*, by Stanley Klein.

The parent who finds that he or she disagrees with the school "M" team's evaluation of the child may request, in writing, that another evaluation be performed. Parents are also entitled to ask for an independent evaluation, or one that is conducted by a qualified examiner who is not affiliated with the agency or school responsible for the decision. Such an independent evaluation may be at public expense. However, if a hearing has already been held and the judgment has been that the school's evaluation is appropriate, the independent evaluation cannot be paid for by public funds. The results of such a private evaluation must be considered by the school, and may be presented as evidence at any hearings which may follow.

INDIVIDUALIZED EDUCATION PLAN (IEP)

The IEP is a critical element in P.L. 94-142. It is both the mechanism for providing that educational plans are tailored to the specific needs of the child and the means for parents to participate in developing these plans. The IEP is "that part of the new law which gives parents an equal voice in the educational program given to their children."[6] Parents are to be included in the process of writing a child's IEP, and the school is required to have the parents' written consent to carry out the plan.

What exactly is an IEP? It is a written document to be individualized to the needs of a single child, rather than to a class or group of children. The special education to be provided is to be specifically designed to meet the child's needs. The program should be fully explained in writing and not be just in outline form.

Five major items are to be included in an IEP.

1. A statement of the child's present levels of educational performance
2. A statement of annual goals for the child, including short-term educational objectives
3. A statement of specific educational and related services (physical therapy, occupational therapy, transportation, etc.) and the extent to which the child will participate in regular classes and activities

4. The anticipated dates for the beginning of these services and the length of time they will be provided
5. Concrete ways that the short-term objectives will be evaluated

The IEP is the cornerstone for assuring that the educational plan developed for each child will in fact address his individual needs. Every child with a handicap is required by P.L. 94-142 to have an IEP written for him. In the planning of the child's IEP, the parent has the opportunity, and the responsibility, to be an active participant in the child's educational program.

Parents are to be included in IEP planning meetings, and at later meetings held to review or revise the child's IEP. Other participants in IEP meetings, as outlined in the law, are to be: the child's teacher; a representative of the school or agency (other than the teacher) who is qualified in special education; the child, if appropriate; and other individuals at the discretion of the parent or the agency. This means that parents can bring to the meeting a person whom they feel knows the child or can help to represent the child's needs.

Some parents may find that it is difficult to express their own convictions about the child's needs in the presence of "experts" who seem to be very glib in their use of professional jargon and data. Parents do need to remember that they, by virtue of their lengthy day-to-day experience with the child, are the real experts on how that child learns and reacts to new situations. This knowledge is crucial to a successful IEP. The best IEPs represent a meeting of professional knowledge with the child's unique needs and personality. It is this knowledge of the child as a unique individual that the parent must bring to the IEP meeting.

Parents can ask school personnel to explain any terms that they do not understand. There is no need to feel embarrassed about not knowing what technical terms mean. The parents have the right, and the responsibility, to understand what they are consenting to. "Please explain that to me in different words" can be said in a friendly and tactful manner.

Parents will feel more confident at an IEP meeting if they have done some preparation. Noting, in writing, the main areas that the parent thinks the child needs attention in and the child's strengths and weaknesses will help parents to prevent forgetting important points. Parents can also familiarize themselves with the child's file and previous test results to back up requests that they make.

P.L. 94-142 assures parents that they have the right to inspect, review, and have copies of any records that contain information on their child. Requests for access to the files should be made in writing, and access must be granted by the agency prior to the IEP meeting. This information may be useful in supporting the parents' case.

Once the IEP is formulated, the parents' written consent is necessary for it to be carried out. Parents should be sure that they have a copy of the IEP and that they have ample time to review and think about it before signing. Questions parents may want to consider include: Does the IEP state the goals and objectives the way that the parent understands them to have been discussed and agreed upon? Are the objectives listed in concrete, rather that general, terms? Are they stated in such a way that they can be measured to determine whether they have been met or not? Are specific dates included for the beginning of the program, and its length?

DUE PROCESS

The law provides a recourse for parents who disagree with the school system, whether that disagreement be about the school's decision in the areas of identification, evaluation, or placement. When discussions with school personnel do not help to settle a dispute in any of these areas, the parent is entitled to request an impartial hearing. The parent should ask for this in writing, and should refer to it as an "impartial hearing." This is not a legal court hearing. The impartial hearing cannot be conducted by any employee of the state or school district or anyone involved with the education or care of the child. This is what makes it "impartial."

Both parents and the school have the following rights at these hearings.

1. To be accompanied and advised by individuals (attorneys or advocates)
2. To present evidence, confront, cross-examine, and compel witnesses
3. To prohibit introduction of evidence not disclosed to the other party at least 5 days prior to the hearing
4. To obtain written recordings of the hearing and of the findings and decisions

Parents who are still dissatisfied after the hearing can appeal further to the State Department of Education. This Department must then conduct its own impartial review of the hearing. This process of hearings and appeals is designed to protect the rights of children and parents. It is the mechanism by which parents can, if they need to, complain publicly to get the school system to do what it should.

Parents who are considering the hearing and appeal process will want to read further on these subjects. (See Appendix B, Education. The booklet "How to Prepare for a Due Process Hearing," available from the Coordinating Council for Handicapped Children in Chicago, for example, has helpful suggestions and sample dialogues which may be useful in planning effective ways for parents to state opinions and counter opposition.)

OTHER ALTERNATIVES

The intent of P.L. 94-142 is that each child shall be provided with an education appropriate to his needs. For some children with highly specialized needs, a program offered in a private school may, in fact, be the one most suitable. A "free, appropriate education" may be a placement of the child by the state or local school district in a private setting. The state maintains its obligation to pay for the child's education, but it contracts with the private agency to provide what it cannot.

Residential schools may be considered by parents because of special needs of the child. Even to consider a residential school placement may seem anachronistic in this era of the thrust toward mainstreaming. But residential schools do exist and parents may want to investigate them.

Consideration of a residential school means weighing the advantages of the program offered over the advantages of the child remaining at home with the family. The first question should be: "What does the child *really* need?" Then parents can think about *where* the child can get what he needs and where compromises can be made. Just because something is not available in the local school district does not mean that it cannot be made available.

Thinking about residential placement raises painful issues for families. Parents may ask themselves, "Is this rejection? Am I an inadequate parent — a failure — to this child? How will I know if the program is good for the child and if the child is happy or unhappy?" In addition to the parents' doubts or guilt, other children in the family will have their own reactions. Some may wonder, "If I am sick (or bad) will I be sent away too?" The possibility of such a placement needs to be explored openly and fully with all family members.

THE CHILD'S EDUCATION IN PERSPECTIVE

There is no denying that the child's educational experience is a vitally important part of that child's life and development. Parents have a greater stake in educational decisions than the school does, for the family must live, day by day, with the results of those decisions. But decisions about educational placements are not necessarily permanent. They can be reviewed, reassessed, and changed if they are not working out well for the child.

Parents will want to keep an eye on the child's educational progress, just as they do with their other children. Communication with the child's teacher needs to be maintained so that potential problems can be discussed before they seem to be hopeless to either parent or teacher. Parents and teachers each have vital perspectives and viewpoints on the child and his needs. If parents and teachers can see themselves as mutually respected partners in working with the child, the child can only benefit.

The education of the child is but one piece, albeit an important one, in the overall life of the family. The family is composed of a number of individuals, each of whom has his or her own needs for growth and development. The family needs continually to seek a balance of these needs so that any one person's do not overshadow those of the others for long periods of time.

QUESTIONS FOR PARENTS

1. Is my child receiving the education and support services that I feel he or she needs?
2. Do I have information (tests and assessments) on my child on which to base my opinions as to what he needs educationally?
3. Do I understand that these tests have limitations and are best used as guides to understanding the child?
4. Do my fears about my child being in a regular school stem from my desire to protect him?
5. Can I discuss my concerns about my child's school experience freely with his teacher?
6. Can I listen to the teachers viewpoint before I react emotionally?
7. Do I understand what my child's rights are under P.L. 94-142?
8. Do I understand what my options are if I disagree with the school's recommendations?
9. Do I know where to find more information, and help, in securing my child's rights?

REFERENCES

1. Brewer, Garry D. and Kakalik, James S, *Handicapped Children: Strategies for Improving Services*, McGraw-Hill, 1979.
2. Pendler, Betty, When Is a Child Ready for Mainstreaming, *The Exceptional Parent*, October 1979.
3. Lusthaus, Charles and Lusthaus, Evelyn, When is a Child Ready for Mainstreaming, *The Exceptional Parent*, October 1979.
4. Blatt, Burton, When is a Child Ready for Mainstreaming, *The Exceptional Parent*, October 1979.

5. Dean, Dorothy; Klein, Stanley D., Ed., in *Psychological Testing of Children, A Consumer's Guide,* Exceptional Parent Press, 1977.
6. Adams, Howard, A Parent's Guide to the Education for All Handicapped Children Act, available from the Spina Bifida Association of Greater Kansas City, P.O. Box 5462, Kansas City, Missouri 64131.

8
ISSUES OF MIDDLE CHILDHOOD
The Years from 6 to 12

Families may experience the years of middle childhood in very different ways. For many families, these years represent a time of relative peace. Parents have survived the battles of acceptance of what is. Often, the worst of the struggles to find care and treatment for the child are over, and decisions about his educational placement are made. Parents have had time to grow to love the child and are able to find joy and pride in his accomplishments. The storms and upheavals of adolescence have not yet begun. The temptation for many parents is to "take a breather," and not to look ahead to the issues that lie in wait. The questions about the child's life as an adult — opportunities for jobs, housing, sex, and marriage — are placed aside. This need to withdraw for a time from confrontation with the issues, although it may be frustrating to the organizers of parent groups, may be necessary for the individual family to restore its sense of balance and perspective.

Other families find the years of middle childhood quite different. For, as some things become easier with time; others become more difficult. The experience of watching a child endure pain is one that is likely to become harder, not easier, for the parents each time it happens. Parents of children who undergo repeated surgical procedures may find that their own reactions to these events become more intense. The child with a physical disability is also becoming bigger and heavier, and including him or her in all the usual family errands and outings becomes more cumbersome. Some favorite family pastimes — skiing, or hiking — may become difficult if not impossible for the whole family to do together.

The reality of the disability and what it means in concrete terms are becoming more apparent. Parents may come to a painful awareness of the fact that their jobs as parents do not decrease at this age as they do with other children. This child continues to be more dependent on parental help, whether it be with toileting, dressing, ambulation, or the need for supervision.

Society's reactions to children with disabilities are likely to seem very different to parents as the child grows closer to adolescence. The young child on crutches may have been seen as "cute." (The success of the use of young children as "poster children" attests to the validity of the appeal of the small child, patronizing though it may be.) But as the child approaches his teens, he is no longer as easily viewed as cute. Behaviors that were tolerated or even approved of in young children are not any longer. The child's awkwardness or developmental lags may be more painfully visible, especially outside the home.

The years from 6 to 12 are, for children, usually a time when the emphasis is on learning, mastery, and developing a sense of independence. The child builds a sense of self and self-esteem through repeatedly mastering new skills and new areas of knowledge. These are usually the years of experimentation with sports, clubs, and music lessons. Some children "specialize" and develop extensive collections and knowledge of stamps, or model cars, or insects. Children learn more about responsibility as they are assigned chores at home or take over the care of the family pets. Relationships with peers become much more important, and how things are going with a best friend or "buddy" may have a great deal to do with how a child is feeling.

All of these areas have relevance for the child with a disability, although the time at which they become important may have more to do with developmental age than chronological age, and the approaches to them may differ as the specific disability is accomodated to.

The family as a whole may have a somewhat different focus during these years as well. Qeustions about the overall style of life of this family become issues to be considered. Where will the family live, and how will it use its leisure time? How can the needs of the child be balanced against the needs of the other people in the family, including those of the parents? Each family answers these questions for itself, whether it does so with conscious thought and planning or by default.

LEARNING AND MASTERY

The development of learning and the mastering of skills and subject matter are important contributors to the child's emerging sense of his or her worth as a person. Of course, the specific things that a child is learning at any given time will vary enormously, depending upon the developmental age, the disability, and his or her abilities and interests. For the child who is retarded, feelings of self-worth and competence may grow as he masters yet another small step in dressing himself or in helping a parent with a chore. The child in a wheelchair may need to explore many crafts and hobbies before he finds one that he cares about doing well in. Any child needs to experience success, even though he will also have failures, in order to feel pride in his accomplishments.

Being successful requires that appropriate goals have been set. If we have expected far too much of ourselves, we will feel disappointed with a reasonable amount of progress. We will still have fallen short of our goal. The establishment of reasonable goals for a child with a disability can be a difficult matter for parents. The child's interests and abilities are still being discovered. Sometimes, they lie in unexpected places. Some areas of difficulty may first show up during these years of middle childhood.

Some problems, such as learning disabilities or perceptual difficulties, may not be apparent until the child is challenged by certain kinds of learning in school. Many parents of children with spina bifida and hydrocephalus, for example, are dismayed to learn that the child has hand-eye coordination problems or learning difficulties in addition to the things they were already dealing with.

The parent whose child has not received a clear diagnosis of his problems has an especially difficult time in attempting to decide what is a reasonable goal for the child. There may be quite genuine confusion as to whether a particular area is difficult for the child because he does not have the ability to master it at this time or whether it is because of unwillingness or a lack of motivation. Parents may place undue emphasis on a particular skill to allay their own fears. They may think, "If he can do this, I can be reassured about his potential" or, "If he can't do this, my fears are justified." Thus the mastery of tasks which would otherwise be seen as quite ordinary becomes weighted with major implications.

As parents watch a child struggle to master a task, whether it be buttoning his clothes or playing the piano, their own feelings and wishes for him are aroused. It is hard to watch a child struggle with things that seem to come easily to other children. Unresolved feelings of anger about the unfairness of disabilities in children may make it difficult to achieve any sort of objectivity about the child's efforts. Parents are torn between their wishes for the child and their fear that they will allow the child to settle for less than he can be. These conflicting feelings lead to inconsistency, with the parent sticking to high expectations one day and abandoning them the next.

To eliminate much of the confusion, both parent and child need to be in agreement as to what the goal is in a particular task. Parents may wish to consult with the child's teachers and therapists to obtain information on what these people think is a reasonable goal for this particular child at this particular time. Next, the task needs to be broken down into its component parts and analyzed. This is particularly important for the child who is retarded, who may need to concentrate on small steps. Tasks such as hand-washing and dressing have many steps and may be overwhelming in their entirety. The child with a physical disability may need modifications in some steps. A rolling serving cart on wheels or an attachment to a wheelchair may enable the child to carry dishes or equipment from one place to another.

For the child to take pride in mastering an activity, he must feel that he has actually accomplished something. Parental approval is one way that the child is able to know when he has succeeded. Most parents realize the importance of giving the child credit and praising him for successful efforts. But how that praise is worded and delivered can have important implications.

Effective praise needs to be specific to the task at hand. "You did a nice job of setting the table" tells the child something about the job that he has done. "Oh, what wonderful boy!" does not. Praise worded in this way does not allow the child to take pride in what he has done but becomes a much more global statement about what he *is*. If a child is consistently told that he is good when he succeeds, he may logically assume that he is equally bad when he fails. Not doing well at a particular task can feel to the child more like not being a good person. If the child hears instead, "You were doing OK until you got to this part," he will be more able to continue to work on the task without feeling that he is a failure.

The child needs to feel that what he has done is good because it is really good, not because the person who did it is disabled. Praise cannot be indiscriminate. The child is very likely to know perfectly well when an effort is sloppy and the praise is hollow. Ideally, every child would find at least one area or activity in which he could be genuinely capable and receive respect not only from his family but from others. Finding this activity for a child who is dsiabled may be challenging for parents. It may take considerable effort and experimentation with different hobbies and crafts. Music, art, woodworking, collections, photography, nature, and the like are all possible avenues to explore. Finding a hobby or area that truly interests the child will not only allow him to develop mastery but also provide him with interests that can be pursued in later life and provide access to friendships with groups of people who share these interests.

INDEPENDENCE

The years of middle childhood are typically a time when rapid strides toward independence are made. Parents of nondisabled children may in fact feel that they are continually restraining their child's insistence that he can go off by himself and that he does not need supervision. The child with a disability, on the other hand, does not have the same opportunities to try out his wings. He may not only be restricted by the effects of the disability, but he may also be further confined by the necessity to carry out prescribed exercises, care, and routines.

Fostering the child's sense of independence is critical, both for the short run, so that he will need less assistance in school, and for the long run, so that he can continue to develop the ability to manage his own life as much as possible. Promoting independence may require conscious thought. It may be easier, on a day-to-day basis, to do "for" the child. Stepping aside and allowing the child to struggle and experiment may seem less natural than helping him, but it is essential.

A sense of independence comes about in two major ways. The first of these is the gradual taking over by the child of aspects of his own care. Although the child may continue to need help in some areas, such as in putting on braces, he or she may be quite able to take over the other steps that come before and after. The other major way that independence is developed is through the experience of being apart from the parents — at school, at friends' houses, at camp — and by learning to make choices and decisions on his own.

Some accomodations may need to be made in the household and its routines to allow the child with a disability to assume more responsibility for his own care. Some of the areas parents may want to consider include the following.

1. Are the things that the child needs accessible and convenient? Perhaps the clothing rod in the child's closet needs to be lowered so that he can reach the hangers from a wheelchair. Are the items he or she needs in the bathroom within reach? Perhaps open shelves would be more convenient than cupboards; or the cabinet below the sink could be removed to allow space for a stool or a wheelchair. Is a mirror placed so that the child can easily see it for grooming?

2. Does the child have the necessary skills? Does he know, for example, how to transfer safely from his bed to a wheelchair? Parents who are concerned about the child's ability to perform transfers or who are unsure about how to teach him these skills may want to consult with a physical therapist.

3. Are items of clothing selected both for their appearance and for their ease in putting on and removing? Fasteners, for example, should be located where the child can reach them and constructed so

that the child can open and close them readily when he needs to use the toilet. Does the child go to the store with the parent and participate in choosing colors and styles of clothing? The experience of shopping contains many lessons in independence. The child can learn to handle and spend money, to make decisions, and to live with the results of those decisions. The child may need to learn through trial and error that an attractive sweater may be uncomfortable to put on or made of a scratchy fabric.

4. Does the child take some responsibility for his own exercises and routines? Schedules of exercises that have been prescribed for the child are rarely things that he likes or wants to do. It is almost impossible for a child to grasp the long-term benefits of daily exercises. The parent may become the "bad guy" who nags at the child each day. One way that parents can extricate themselves from this position is to increase communication between the professional involved and the child. If an orthopedic surgeon has prescribed exercises, for example, the parent can ask that the doctor talk directly to the child, looking him in the eye and explaining what needs to be done and why. This helps to make clear to the child that these tedious routines are not something that the parents dreamed up. The child will perhaps begin to see that there is a pay-off for him, even though it may be in the distant future.

While the parent may need to initiate routines and help the child as he learns how to carry them out and how to fit them into the day's activities, the responsibility should gradually become the child's. The child in a wheelchair can be taught to do push-ups, to change his position, and to use a mirror to inspect his own skin for pressure areas. Most children during these years become more modest about exposing their bodies, even to parents. This can be a powerfully motivating force for the child to learn to do his more private care by himself. When the parent *must* help, protecting the child's modesty as much as possible with clothing or towels will convey a sense of respect for him or her as a separate, independent person.

5. Does the child have enough time allotted to carry out self-care? Frustration and a sense of failure are likely to result if the child feels pressured by time and worries that he will not be able to complete his tasks. Perhaps his alarm clock needs to be set one-half hour earlier while he is practicing a new part of self-care; or the family may need to reschedule each person's allotted time for use of the bathroom. Other family members can do in their bedrooms the things that don't require water, such as dressing, hair curling, or applying makeup.

6. Is the child expected to contribute a fair share of effort to the household functioning? Is he or she assigned chores on a regular basis? In order for participation in chores to be meaningful, the task

must be "real." It must actually be something that the family needs to have done. It also must be done consistently. To be sure, the task needs to be tailored to the child's abilities. Often some accomodations must be made. A rolling cart or a worktable at the right height can allow a physically disabled child to set the table or perform sedentary jobs like polishing silver, making sandwiches, and the like. The child who needs supervision and direction can work with a parent on tidying up a room, dusting, or performing simple cooking tasks. The child who needs an excessive amount of help also needs to learn that he can give help, whether that be carrying wastebaskets or bringing guests sugar for their tea.

Independence also requires that the child begin to learn that he can operate away from his parents. The bonds that develop between a child and parents who have struggled with and fought for him can be very, very strong. There is nothing inherently negative about these intense bonds, unless they stifle the child's (or the parent's) opportunities to experience himself as a competent person in other situations and in other relationships. Both children and parents need to learn that the child can safely be away and that other people can help him deal with problems if necessary.

For many children with disabilities, attendance at summer camp programs is a good way to get this experience and to have a wonderful time doing it. Excellent summer camps staffed by people with interest and training in disabilities are available. Many, like those run by state Easter Seal Societies, offer scholarships to those children whose families would have difficulty in paying the fees. Many children who attend regular public schools also find that they make deep and lasting friendships with other children with disabilities while at camp.

Sleeping overnight at a friend's or relative's house is another way to gain some of this experience. Parents may want to foster this by encouraging the child to have friends, both disabled and nondisabled, to sleep over. Sometimes, however, the guests' parents seem reluctant to reciprocate. Parents may find it necessary to do some tactful encouraging and reassuring to other parents who may be fearful about the child's needs or the possibility that he may get hurt. It may not be easy to work the conversation around to the point where the parent can say, "Oh, Johnny doesn't need any special help except for . . . ." Not all people will respond with invitations; but some are likely to.

FRIENDSHIPS

Friendships become increasingly important to children during the years of middle childhood. This can be a frustrating matter for parents, who are not able to arrange and schedule visits with friends as they used to.

When children are younger, parents plan and organize visits with playmates; they do the telephoning, the transporting, and the supervision of play. As nondisabled children get older, they increasingly arrange their own activities and are likely to go off on their bikes or to the movies without thinking of their friend who is disabled.

Parents are left with more indirect methods of operating. The parent can encourage the child to be more active in telephoning friends and inviting them over; but the child who is shy about being "different" may see this as pushing and become resentful. Parents can try to see that the house is an attractive place for children to be, with snacks and activities available; but many parents have mixed feelings at best about the time and energy this may take. Not every parent wishes the house to become the neighborhood "drop-in" center.

The approach of adolescence is likely to be a difficult time for children with disabilities. This is an age in which it is extremely important for most children not to seem to be different. Nondisabled youngsters may fret about their appearance, their body size and shape, and whether they have the "right" brands of tennis shoes and jeans. Children who are engrossed in their own struggles to be just like the rest of the group can be quite limited in their awareness of or thoughtfulness about other differences.

Children with disabilities are unique individuals and will have varying responses to these stresses. Some children who have been through experiences of pain and surgery seem to evolve a more mature sense of values than their peers. They are able to pay more attention to someone's feelings than to his brands of clothing. But all children are likely to have moments of tears and hurt when they feel rejected by their peers. Parents may suffer, too, as they try to comfort. It helps to remember that *all* adolescents, whether disabled or not, go through times of feeling that their bodies are ugly and that they have no friends. These feelings are not specific to children with disabilites; they are part of living with a changing body and a growing awareness of others.

What can parents do to help the child through this period? The first and most important thing for the parent to do is to get rid of the assumption that the child is suffering or is rejected solely because he is disabled. This assumption leads nowhere but to anger, resentment, or pity, none of which will help the child. While it may be true that a few people are so uncomfortable that they cannot deal with the child who is disabled, the parent who jumps to the conclusion that most people are that way closes many doors to the child.

For the child to have friends, he must know something about *being* a friend. He must know something about sharing, about listening, about participating with enthusiasm, and about sensitivity to the needs of others. These are not qualities that develop quickly; most people continue to grow in these areas all of their lives. But it is hoped that the child will have had some successful experiences with friends in earlier years to draw on. The child who interprets all slights as deliberate rejections may need to be gently reminded that perhaps some other explanations are possible. Maybe his classmates are *not* looking down on him because of the disability. Perhaps some of them feel shy, too. Has the child noticed anyone who looks lonely in the lunchroom or at recess that he could be friendly to?

Parents can help to see to it that the child looks and dressed well. As much as the family budget will allow, the child's clothing should be as stylish as possible. The child needs to be taught to attend to haircombing, clean fingernails, toothbrushing, and the like. This can be a delicate situation for the disabled or retarded child who is trying to learn to be neat on his own; parents want to encourage without being insulting. The truth is, however, that an unkempt appearance accentuates the difference of a disability. As Carol Michaelis writes, "First impressions count. Very few people give the disabled person a second chance."[1]

The child who has a more serious but more easily understood disability, such as paralyzed legs, may actually have an easier time being accepted by his schoolmates than the child with a more "minor" disability. The children who are on the fringe — who have learning disabilities or mild brain damage or retardation — may have a harder time of it during these years because their friends are confused by the fact that they look quite "normal."

All parents of children with disabilities are likely to experience hurt and pain as they watch the child struggling to cope with rejection. The old urges to protect the child may surge forward, and parents may wish to keep the child within the family or transfer him to a more protected school setting. But the child will not be as able to cope with the nondisabled world as an adult unless he or she has had some experience with this in childhood. In Verda Heisler's words, "The pain of occasional cruelty of other children is *less* harmful than the pain of segregation from the peer world."[2]

PSYCHOLOGICAL DEVELOPMENT

Some time during these middle years of childhood, the child is likely to confront a new awareness of his own disability. The younger child is more likely to harbor assumptions like, "When I get bigger I'll get stronger too." At some point, the child will realize that this is not so. Parents may not always be immediately aware that this is happening. Sometimes, it is the experience of watching a much younger sibling or neighbor's child learn to toddle and walk that shocks the child into realizing that he *is* bigger and he *can't* walk.

Children can become depressed. It may be difficult for parents to differentiate between natural periods of sadness or anger about the disability and deeper depression that comes about when the child generalizes the unacceptability of his disability to his whole self. When this happens, the child feels that he is worthless as a person. Keeping the lines of communication open, so that the child can talk freely, will help parents to distinguish between natural periods of sadness and longer-lasting, more generalized feelings of worthlessness.

Withdrawal is a rather common occurrence in physically disabled children. Children who cannot use physical activity as a "safety valve" for pent up feelings have fewer choices when they feel that they cannot cope. Withdrawing into silence or passive TV watching may seem to be the only recourse.

The child who has little control over his body or what happens to it — who is repeatedly subjected to medical examinations, hospitalizations, or painful procedures — may feel that he has very few areas in his life that he can control. Sometimes, a slowing down in school work or failure to do assignments can be a form of rebellion. The child may be saying, "I may not have control over what happens to me, but I *can* control when my homework is done!" The child who shows this pattern can be assisted not only by extra help in structuring his school work but also by more opportunity to express his feelings and assume control over other parts of his life. Parents can allow the child to make more choices and show respect for his wishes and opinions, even when they disagree.

When a child consistently misbehaves, it may be necessary for parents to step back and take a more analytical look at the situation. Although some behaviors that are disturbing to parents may have their origins in the disability, even these can become exaggerated or habitual. The parent needs to consider: What is it that the child hopes to *gain* from the behavior? Behaviors, and misbehaviors, are purposeful. As Lawrence Zuckerman and Michael Yura point out, "One of the most crucial concepts that we need to understand is that children's misbehavior is purposeful. It is no accident that children consistently exhibit the same misbehavior."[3] These authors suggest that problem behaviors may stem from four "mistaken" goals of the child.

1. Attention. If the child feels, "I only count when I am noticed," this need will be overwhelming and it will matter less whether the attention is positive or negative. The important thing will be to be noticed.

2. Power. Power struggles may develop between parents and children. Usually, the child who fights for power is tying to shore up his own sense of self-importance. Underneath, he may feel weak and insecure.
3. Revenge. This is more extreme; when a child wants revenge, he feels that there is no hope of acceptance and that his only option is to hurt back.
4. Inadequacy. The child who feels inadequate is sure that he will fail before he tries, so that there is no point in trying to behave well or to please others.

Each of these underlying motivations has important implications for the ways that parents can act to change the child's behaviors. Parents who wish further help in dealing with a child's problem behaviors may want to read *Raising the Exceptional Child: Meeting the Everyday Challenges of the Handicapped or Retarded Child* by Zuckerman and Yura.[3] Professional assistance may also help by providing an objective viewpoint, additional information for problem-solving, and support for parents as they deal with their own uncertainty and guilt.

In order to understand themselves, children need to understand their disability. Children need factual, honest information about their disabilities from a very early age. Many people who work with disabled teenagers express surprise at how little many of these adolescents seem to know about their bodies and their disabilities. It is easy for parents to forget that all the information they have struggled to obtain may not have been translated and communicated to the child, or to remember that the child may harbor distorted versions of what doctors have told the parents.

Parents should not wait for the child to ask; some children will not. Early information about the disability can be simple, much as early information about sex is handled. It is important to also tell the child, in most cases, something about the cause of the disability or how it happened. If parents can discuss freely and matter-of-factly both how the child's body is like most peoples' and how it is different, children can be more matter of fact about their questions.

Parents may have difficulty doing this because they worry about revealing their own feelings to the child. The child may be very reassured by the parent who says, "Sometimes I feel sad that you can't run," or "I feel bad when you have to go to the hospital." Think of it from the child's point of view: how strange and puzzling it would be to have parents who remained calm, cheerful and stoical while you experienced pain, fear, and frsutration! It is not necessary or desirable for parents to weep and wail or be hysterical in front of their children, simply to say honestly that they do have feelings about what is happening.

THE FAMILY AS A WHOLE

Once a family is past the stage of adding new members and is no longer caught up in the care of babies, issues of what kind of life the family will lead become important. Sometimes, families remain so engrossed in the care of the disabled child and with worries about his health or his future that they neglect to consider the overall balance of their lives. In the long run, the child will not benefit from remaining the focus of the family's worry and concern. He will do better if he lives in a family in which each member is alive and vibrant and has an equal opportunity to grow and develop.

The years of middle childhood may be the time when problems stemming from the long-term effects of stress begin to appear. The ways in which people deal with acute stress or crises are not necessarily the best ways to deal with long-term anxieties or worries. For example, many parents manage to cope with a child's serious illness or major surgery by becoming "strong and silent." They may submerge their own fears and grief in order to be available and strong for the child. This may be an excellent way to manage during a crisis, but may not serve as well if it becomes imbedded as a permanent, prevailing way of deiling with life.

Each of the parents faces his or her own individual needs at different stages of life. For men, these years may be a time when they have reached a desired level of competence or achievement in work. And yet, they may feel that they cannot fully provide for all the needs, and the extras, of the people in the family as they wish. Difficult choices about financial expenditures must still be made. The family may still need to rely on financial assistance to meet the needs. Many parents *do* feel trapped into taking or staying in jobs they dislike because of better pay or better insurance benefits. At this point in life, both men and women may confront the realization that they may not fulfill their own highest dreams or ambitions. The process of acceptance of self goes on throughout adulthood.

Many women who have opted to remain at home during their children's early years would, ordinarily, begin to think about looking outward, developing interests, and taking jobs when their children enter school. Mothers of children with disabilities may feel cheated of these options if the child still needs assistance, supervision, and frequent trips to clinics. Others feel forced into working when they do not wish to in order to help meet the financial demands.

Other children in the family are growing, too, and have their own needs to branch out on their own. They may have many feelings of guilt about the things they can do that their brother or sister cannot, or of resentment at the demands placed on them to help out. Siblings can cope much better with the needs of the disabled family member if they believe, deep down, that their own needs and wishes are farily taken into account.

Brothers and sisters may have their own misperceptions about the disability. They may worry about what caused it, or be afraid of becoming sick or disabled themselves. They need to be included in the family's struggles, to share in discussions about what is happening, and to be allowed to accompany the child to the hospital and participate in the experiences. They need accurate, honest information — using the correct words, such as "retardation" or "brain damage" — both for their own acceptance and so that they will be able to handle the questions of their own friends matter-of-factly.

Family members need to share both the pain and the joys of living. The family needs rest, relaxation, and fun. The family that feels so overwhelmed by and preoccupied with the stress that it cannot incorporate "play" into its life may benefit from counseling aimed at exploring new ways of coping and changing the balance of the family.

QUESTIONS FOR PARENTS

1. Do I have a clear idea of what is reasonable in setting goals for my child?
2. Can I recognize the role my own hopes and fears play in setting goals?
3. Does my child have ample opportunity to experience success?
4. Is my child doing as much for himself as he could be?
5. How can I make this more possible? Do I need to step aside so he can try, or do we need to make modifications in the house or the routines?
6. Can I encourage my child to develop friendships?
7. Can I let my child be without me, at camp or at a friend's house?
8. Does my child look as neat as he can? Are his clothes as much like those of other children as possible?
9. Have I explained the disability to the child, and to his brothers and sisters? Are they free to ask questions?
10. Is our family able to provide a needed balance of fun and relaxation?

REFERENCES

1. Michaelis, Carol, Why Can't Johnny Look Nice, Too?, *The Exceptional Parent*, April 1979.
2. Heisler, Verda, *A Handicapped Child in the Family: A Guide for Parents*, Grune and Stratton, 1972.
3. Zuckerman, Lawrence and Yura, Michael T., *Raising the Exceptional Child: Meeting the Everyday Challenges of the Handicapped or Retarded Child*, Hawthorne Books, 1979.

9
ISSUES OF ADOLESCENCE
Psychosocial Development

Many of the issues already discussed in this book will come back into focus during the years of adolescence. Parents may have dealt with acceptance of the disability or with relationships with friends and relatives; but now, the teenager with a disability must face these questions for him or herself. The old issues are back again, but this time it is the adolescent with the disability who must struggle with them directly. For parents, the old conflict between wanting to encourage and wanting to protect may reappear with new strength. For adolescence means that "the future" is at hand; the child's ability to find his or her place in the world will soon be demonstrated.

It is difficult to make general statements about nondisabled adolescents. Each teen's personality, physical and emotional development, and family and social relationships affect how these years are experienced. It is even more difficult to make general statements about adolescents with disabilities who may, after all, be quite different from each other as well as from their nondisabled peers. The situation of an aggressive, outgoing, determined girl with cerebral palsy may be very different from that of a shy, introverted boy who is blind.

However, some predictable events and issues arise during adolescence. Parents and professionals who are involved with adolescents with disabilities can think about and consider these issues. Then, they can consider how the unique personality and abilities of the individual teenager affects the resolution of these questions. The physical changes associated with the attainment of sexual maturity are the basis of one such group of issues. Questions about what approaching adulthood means — in terms of living arrangements, employment, intimate relationships, and recreation — will arise and will need to be struggled with.

These are difficult and complex questions for both teenagers and parents. They tap our deepest hopes, fears, and beliefs. The values we hold in relation to independence, marriage, sex, and the very meaning of life may affect our responses to the teenager's situation. As parents, or as professionals working with teenagers with disabilities, we may have to reexamine our priorities and our ideas about what is most important in life. Our own life goals may not "fit" for our children. We may need to be open to the possibility that different goals may be just as valuable.

Approaching adulthood means looking beyond the immediate family to the larger community about us. This may mean confronting the fears, inadequacies, and injustices that exist in the world in a way that was perhaps less necessary when the child could be more sheltered within the family. It can be a cruel shock to discover that the facilities and opportunities that a disabled person needs are not available, and that the rest of the world does not share any sense of urgency in making them available. Social change takes time. This is why it is essential for parents of young children to look around, see what is needed, and become involved. Attitudinal changes and needed programs can be achieved, but this is not likely to happen spontaneously. Social change comes from social pressure; and social pressure comes from the combined efforts of committed, active people.

What are the major issues that arise during adolescence? To this writer, they seem to fall into four main areas: the teenager's self-concept; relationships with peers; formulating life goals; and the question of leaving home. Each of these areas encompasses a variety of questions which will have a profound impact on how the adolescent moves towards adulthood. Each is worthy of careful thought on the part of those who are involved with the teenager with a disability.

SELF-CONCEPT

One of the most important developmental tasks of adolescence is the matter of coming to an understanding and acceptance of the question, "Who am I?" This involves becoming aware of one's strengths and weaknesses, one's physical body, and one's beliefs and values. Most nondisabled teenagers experience periods of great frustration with their physical appearance and conflicts with parents as they struggle to establish their own values and goals. The questions and issues are no less real for adolescents with disabilities. The struggles may be experienced differently; but how they are manifested may be perfectly "normal" for the maturation of someone with that disability, even though it may look quite different from what one would expect from a teenager who does not have a disability.

Most disabling conditions do not affect physical and hormonal maturation in any significant way. Boys and girls with disabilities will develop body hair and the other manifestations of sexual maturity. For some disabling conditions, such as spina bifida, the tendency may be toward experiencing these changes at a somewhat earlier age than "average." This means that parents not only cannot delay the discussion of menstruation or other sexual changes with their children, but in some cases must also be prepared to deal with these questions early.

Thus the adolescent with a physical disability must deal not only with the changes in his or her own body but also with the fact that in some ways that body is not like most other teenagers. For some, this means giving up childhood fantasies that someday the problem will be "outgrown"; that paralyzed legs will get stronger or that small stature will get bigger. Such teenagers may need to go through their own sadness, grief, and anger. It may be very painful for parents to watch a child grieve for what cannot be. The most helpful response for the child, however, may be, "It's all right to feel sad that your legs will not let you dance or ski like other kids." These expressions of sorrow and grief on the part of the teenager with a disability may reactivate the parent's own sadness. There is nothing wrong with a parent saying to the child, "Sometimes I feel sad about that too." On the contrary, this sharing of feelings may help the child to express and deal with his or her own feelings and pave the way for greater acceptance of the reality. The adolescent who feels that he or she cannot express or acknowledge sad or angry feelings may carry those feelings into adulthood in a less open and more destructive way.

The adolescent may become aware of the reality of his or her disability in a new way. The growing awareness of the outside world and the wish to be "just like" other teenagers may bring the disability into sharper focus. For those with retardation, this may be the time that the awareness of being "different" may really strike. The awareness may have been present for some time, but the word that the rest of the world uses — "retarded" — may not have been used openly with the child. Both parents and professionals may experience great difficulty in discussing retardation matter-of-factly with the retarded young person.

This understandable wish to protect the child who is retarded, however, can leave the child both angry and defenseless when it comes to handling the comments or taunts of other children in school or in the neighborhood. Children and young people need to know that they have more trouble than others in learning or remembering certain kinds of things, and that the word which is used to describe this difficulty is called "retardation." They may also need to be reminded about their strengths and encouraged to take pride in the things they can accomplish.

Teenagers with physical disabilities need to know about how bodies work and what, specifically, is different about their own bodies. People who work with teenagers often say that, as a group, they seem to have a poor understanding of what their physical situation is or what treatments their bodies have received. There seems to be, in some young people, a tendency to avoid thinking about things that are painful or frightening. Thus the child may have learned not to think about or to ask questions about his or her bodily functions. Teenagers with disabilities may actually ignore the parts of their bodies that do not work. On a practical level, this may seriously interfere with the formation of a self-concept that includes both strengths and limitations.

The teenager needs to understand the specifics about his or her physiological condition and what treatments he or she is receiving. The young person who does not know these things cannot expect to begin to deal with medical professionals on his or her own, or to take over areas like skin care or bowel and bladder functioning. The ability to look at and care for one's own body, including those parts which are "different," is necessary also for the eventual acceptance of that body as part of oneself.

A sense of sureness and confidence about one's own self-concept also comes in part from increasing independence: being able successfully to take care of oneself and to manage in the world. This, of course, is a theme that runs through the child's entire development. Adolescence is a good time for parents to reevaluate their child's progression toward independence. Are the parents still doing things for the child because it is easier or faster, or because of habit? Is the child learning, as much as possible, to care for clothing, food, and physical needs? Is there ample opportunity to practice making decisions? Does the child have the chance to manage some sums of money independently, and to decide about when to do homework or chores?

It may take special planning and attention to counteract feelings of failure and inadequacy. Some disabilities, such as minimal brain dysfunction, tend to interfere with a variety of learning and activities. Children with these disabilities may have become accustomed to thinking of themselves as clumsy, or inept, or even stupid. As Ernest Siegel says, "By the time the minimally brain-dysfunctioned adolescent enters junior or senior high school, he has experienced repeated failure — socially, academically, or both."[1] In order for the teenager to be able to see and appreciate what he or she can do well, or do better than the last time, praise and encouragement from others are needed.

But the adolescent will not believe statements which are too general: "You are such a wonderful boy," for example. Rather, the praise should be very specific. "You folded the laundry very neatly today" or "This math paper has fewer mistakes than yesterday's" are statements that the adolescent may believe because they are specific and tangible.

Many adolescents need to learn that they can confront their parents, disagree with them, and fight for their own opinions and desires. The experience of handling disagreements within a relationship that maintains an overall element of caring and respect can contribute a great deal to the adolescent's knowledge of himself as a worthwhile person. The ability to disagree with parents, however, requires an increasing sense of oneself as a separate and capable person. It also requires that the parents have a sense of certainty of their own positions and power. It is difficult for parents who are still struggling with guilt or grief to stand firm in their relationships with teenagers. Parents who have not worked through their own guilt or who feel sorry for their children will be more apt to back down or give in when conflicts arise.

Some adolescents with disabilities may have difficulty in being able to disagree with parents in an open and healthy way. If they have undergone painful and frightening hospital experiences in the past, they may have been extremely dependent on the parents' help and support. Or, the adolescent may still need to rely on the parents for help as well as companionship. It may be difficult in such cases to risk losing the good will and support of the parents by challenging their authority. Such teenagers need to learn that asserting their own wishes and opinions is a necessary part of growing up, and that they do not need to sacrifice their parents' respect and good will to do this. The experience of participating in group discussions with other teenagers may be especially helpful in learning to balance self-assertion with respect for others.

The sense of self-esteem that each of us has is strengthened by the knowledge that, in spite of our shortcomings, there are some things that we can do very well. The teenager with a disability may need some help in searching for and developing those strengths and abilities. These satisfactions may be found in a variety of areas: in increasing independence, in hobbies or activities, in school work, or in being a good friend. The teenager may need encouragement to try new activities. Here again, the line between encouragement and coercion may be a difficult one for parents. While some teenagers may eagerly try new hobbies or join new groups, others will be more timid. The older child who is shy needs to retain some degree of choice in what he or she is willing to do. A chance to choose between music lessons or a school interest club may be easier or less threatening than feeling that one has no choice in the face of parental pressure. Some teenagers will respond positively to opportunities to be involved in volunteer or advocacy groups in the community, while others will have their own interests or talents that they prefer to develop.

It is important for the teenager to identify the areas in which he or she is *not* disabled. Cerebral palsy, for example, need not affect one's ability to learn a great deal about history or stamp-collecting. Teenagers who can become acquainted with and enjoy their own individual strengths will experience greater self-esteem. Joyce Slayton Mitchell, speaking to teens in her book, *See Me More Clearly: Career and Life Planning for Teens with Physical Disabilities*, says: "Getting out from under the stereotype — the disability label that others say you are like — is what you have to do. You have to get out of the box that implies you need the same things, have the same joys, have the same fears, need the same education, and go into the same careers as all the others with your particular disability."[2]

RELATIONSHIPS WITH PEERS

Few areas can be as difficult for teenagers with disabilities as that of friendships and social relationships. At the very age when it is most important to fit in and not to be "different," the disability seems to be most conspicuous. Other nondisabled adolescents may be preoccupied with their own struggles and development, and be less than sensitive to the needs and feelings of their classmate with a disability. The teenager with a physical disability may not be able to participate in spur-of-the-moment activities if mobility and transportation require planning and assistance. Teenagers who are unsure of their own abilities and skills may jump to the conclusion that others are reacting to their disability when in fact they are not.

Sometimes, of course, others *are* reacting to the disability. The teenager will probably be much more sensitive to attitudes of others than he or she was in childhood. People with disabilities have been portrayed more often in recent years in movies and television. Often, however, these portrayals emphasize the almost superhuman stoicism, courage, and cheerfulness of people who have succeeded in spite of disabilities. Most adolescents do not wish to be seen as superhumans. They would prefer to be free to be as grumpy, irritable, depressed, or angry as anyone else. As Betty Pieper says to teenagers, "[Being friendly] does not mean that you have to be the stereotype of a 'cheerful cripple.' . . . You do not have any obligation to be cheerful all of the time, or to compensate for your disability by being a wise counselor to everyone else in the world while ignoring your own needs."[3]

In some ways, a disability which is "mild" may present more problems for the adolescent than one which is objectively more severe. Wheelchairs or crutches are fairly easily explained and understood. But adolescents who are mildly retarded or who have minimal brain dysfunction may be able to "pass," or to have their disability not be noticed, in some situations. This may create awkward and difficult questions about when, or if, the teenager needs to say something about the disability. It also may be much harder for other teens to comprehend the existence of a disability which is not obvious but which presents problems in reading, space perception, or the like.

The adolescent with a disability who wishes to have friends will need to learn about *being* a friend, just as all other people do. Learning to initiate conversations, to listen to others, and to show concern for others are essential. Parents may want to help their teenager focus on what he or she has to offer to others. Is it a sense of humor? An ability to help with homework? An interesting hobby to share? The teenager who feels positive about what he or she can contribute to a friendship can be more matter-of-fact about accepting help when it is needed without feeling too dependent.

Feelings of confidence in relationships with others are enhanced when the teenager can feel stylish and attractive. Teens whose disabilities decrease their chances of shopping, clothes-swapping, or make-up experimentation with their peers may need special help in these areas. Parents may need to do some extra coaching in matters of grooming, hair styling, or the use of make-up. Parents may need to be more aware of what clothing is considered stylish by teens, and to lean toward those styles rather than sticking too firmly to their own ideas about what is practical. No longer should parents automatically buy clothes for the youngster and bring them home, as they did when the teen was younger. Even though it may be more cumbersome to take the teenager through clothing stores, the experience of trying on clothes and making choices enhances not only self-esteem but also responsibility and decision-making.

The development of hobbies and skills is especially important during adolescence. Not only do these have the potential for providing hours of satisfaction during adulthood, but they give the teenager something concrete and tangible on which to base contacts with others. It is much easier to strike up conversations with people at a club meeting or an activity than it is to walk (or wheel) into a group of strangers at a party and try to "make friends." It is well worth exploring a wide range of hobbies and activities that may have the potential of stimulating the interest of the adolescent. Art, music, photography, nature or history study, collections of various kinds, crafts, or writing are among the possible areas to explore. Teenagers may need encouragement not to rule out possibilities too quickly. Drama and theater, for example, include a whole range of activities that may appeal to a youngster who initially is shy about being on stage.

Learning to drive is perhaps even more important to a teenager who is disabled than to nondisabled teens. Being able to move about in the world independently can represent a real turning point for the adolescent who feels helpless, dependent, and left out. Modern innovations in adaptive car controls and the availability of driving instruction in the schools for handicapped students mean that driving is now a real possibility for many teenagers with disabilities. Parents and teenagers can inquire about driver education through their local schools. Information on adaptations for cars is available through consumer publications such as "Accent on Living" or local organizations of disabled adults.

LIFE GOALS FOR THE CHILD

Teenagers with disabilities may have a difficult time arriving at career and life goals that are both realistic enough to be within the realm of possibilities and that also allow for full attainment of their potential. They may go through periods of declaring ambitions that seem wildly unrealistic to parents. Nondisabled teenagers may have periods of unrealistic dreams too; but somehow these are not as painful for parents. Parents may have as much trouble settling on realistic goals as does the teenager. The old conflict between wanting the child to excel or succeed and the wish to protect him or her from pain and disappointment may lead the parent to vacillate between wanting too much or too little.

One of the things that teenagers with disabilities need is to be freed from some of the common stereotypes of what people *should* do as adults. They need to grow up knowing that there are more ways than one to live a satisfying adult life. They need to believe truly that not everyone needs to marry or be a parent, and that dignity and respect are to be found in many kinds of jobs and relationships. Parents may have to do some work in exploring their own attitudes and values long before the child approaches adulthood. Stereotypes of family and life styles portrayed in books and on television need to be commented on openly and counteracted. Images of mother, father, and two children in the suburbs can be balanced somewhat by a systematic introduction to a variety of jobs and careers, and to adults with and without disabilities who live alone or with one or more roommates.

Some jobs may be more difficult with particular disabilities. Teenagers, however, should not be too quick to rule out job fields that they are interested in. New ground has been broken in recent years by people with disabilities. There have been, for example, blind people who have graduated from medical school. Before deciding that a particular career is not possible, the teenager and parents should learn as much as they can about what is involved and talk to a variety of people in that field. Then they will be better able to weigh what is required and what modifications might be necessary. Teenagers may need help in learning about jobs and careers in order not to limit their choices too early. Opportunities to learn about different jobs and to observe people working at them will be useful in widening the range of choices and in making realistic decisions.

Job and career choices require a reasonably accurate assessment of abilities and knowledgeable counselors. These may be difficult to find. Many disabilities make accurate testing difficult. Problems with coordination, vision, or learning disabilities, for example, may lead to test results that are distorted in some manner and do not truly reflect the young person's ability. Psychological characteristics — an attitude of "I can't do that," or an unwillingness to take risks or make guesses during testing — can also lead to distorted or inaccurate results. The ideal vocational counselor would be able to be aware of these factors and take them into account, and would also have a far-reaching knowledge about many career areas. He or she would, of course, also possess an abundance of both wisdom and tact in guiding young people toward career decisions. In reality, guidance counselors must deal with demands of heavy workloads and with the impossibility of knowing everything about a particular student or a particular disability. Parents will want to weigh the advice their children are given against their own knowledge and to seek further information when necessary.

As the child with a disability moves into the teenage years, parents may want to reassess the basic skills needed to live or work outside of the parental home. If there are gaps or weaknesses in these skills, they can be worked on and improved. Youngsters who are retarded or who have brain damage may need to have extra attention paid to the kinds of activities they will need to engage in away from home. Ernest Siegel, in his book, *The Exceptional Child Grows Up*, discusses a variety of areas in which the young person may need help.[1] But any child who has needed extra help from parents or other adults may benefit from a fresh look at what he or she can do alone. Areas to evaluate may include: care of self, clothing and belongings; food preparation; use of appliances; and safety precautions. In relation to work, the skills might include using public transportation, following directions, ability to be on time, and the like.

Vocational Rehabilitation Services may be useful in helping to bridge the gap between home and work. Clients accepted by Vocational Rehabilitation may receive diagnosis and evaluation, medical or medically related services, training, income maintenance, and some other services (such as transportation, interpreters or readers, and the like). Not all applicants are accepted; Brewer and Kakalik found that forty-five percent of applications were rejected.[4] Also, there are variations across the country as to what types of disabilities are focused on. The possibility of funding cutbacks on the federal level makes it unlikely that Vocational Rehabilitation departments will be able to expand their services to meet all of the needs. In spite of these facts, however, it is still worthwhile for families to learn about these services and apply for them.

LEAVING HOME

The approaching of the child's 18th birthday, or the time when children are ordinarily expected to leave the nest, may represent a time of crisis for parents. This may well be true whether the child is actually able to go out on his or her own or not. Parents whose children *do* leave — to go to school, or to live on their own — must cope with their own anxieties about how well they will manage without the parent's supervision. They may worry about how the child is caring for his or her health, whether he or she is taking proper care of braces and appliances, and about the possibility of injuries or accidents. The degree of this worrying may lead parents to some painful questioning about just who is the needful one. Does the child need the parent to worry? Or does the parent need the child? As Betty Pendler writes, it may come as a bit of a shock to parents to realize that much of the teaching of self-care to the child is really a preparation for independence and separation.[5]

The process of separating the child's day-to-day life from that of the parents may reveal just how deeply intertwined those lives have become. Parents who have not paid enough attention to themselves as individuals and to each other as lovers and companions as the child was growing up may find it harder to enjoy this new stage in their lives. They may need to become reacquainted with each other and to reexplore their own interests and activities. "Letting go" of the parenting role after such deep involvement may not be easy; it may require a shift in thinking to perceive the rewards and joys of this period of life.

The parent whose child will continue to need care and assistance into adulthood faces a different kind of crisis. "Parents of a child with a severe disability requiring on-going custodial care, monitoring, or support systems realize that their responsibility toward this child is not going to end, but that he will continue to depend on them for the rest of their lives. This recognition comes at a time when many parents are beginning to feel vulnerable anyway."[6]

At a time in life when parents feel the need for some respite, they are again reminded that their responsibilities toward this child will not end as do those of other parents whose children assume total responsibility for themselves. Their parenting job will continue.

Some parents may be quite comfortable having their adult child live with them. Others may feel that even though they themselves are willing to continue to have the child live at home, this would restrict the opportunities for the young adult to experience life more as his or her peers do. Others may genuinely wish for their children to live away from home, but may feel guilty or fearful about these wishes. There are many variations of individual responses to this situation. It is quite normal and usual for the same parents to experience conflicting feelings around these issues. The question is one which calls into play both hopes and fears for the child.

Parents of children who will require some degree of assistance face a number of complexities as they consider possible living arrangements for the child. On the other hand, parents are likely to have mixed feelings about their child's joining a group home or other such living situation. Such a possibility may raise long-dormant guilt about their own wishes to have a placement for the child back when he or she was an infant. It may also mean that parents must face giving up their own roles as protective and nurturing parents. These forces may "pull" the parent toward resisting a move for the child. At the same time, parents may be genuinely fatigued and long for a greater degree of freedom for themselves in their retirement years.

The complexities do not exist only within the family, however. As parents look outward to the community, they discover that society is ambivalent also. The choices of living arrangements for adults who need some help are, in most places, woefully inadequate. While our society gives lip service to ideas of the merits of alternatives such as group homes, much resistance is encountered when such homes are proposed for specific neighborhoods. Fears that people who are disabled may be violent, act out sexually, or otherwise cause problems may be the unspoken reasons for this resistance. In this author's city, the local newspaper quoted a neighborhood resident as saying she opposed a group home near her church because she would be depressed if she saw "those people" when she left her church on Sunday mornings.

The choices become even more limited if parents are searching for a living situation that offers both assistance and a "normalized" life style. Normalization requires that, as is true for the rest of us, different aspects of life are carried out in different places. We generally live in one setting and work in another; we leave our homes for socialization and recreation; we attend classes, churches, and the like in different places. Most adults do not live with "parents," but manage their lives and households alone or in cooperation with other adults in the home. A normalized living setting for people with disabilities provides for these things. It does not require that all aspects of life be based solely on the person's disability or "difference."

Betty Pieper, writing in *Beyond the Family and the Institution: Residential Issues for Today*[7] discusses a number of criteria that families may wish to use when considering living arrangements for their children. Some of her questions include the following.

Did people choose to live here? or were they "placed" like objects?
Do other people of the same age live in similar settings?
Is the residence in a residential neighborhood? Do other people live
     nearby?
Does it have an appearance and address like other homes? (or does it
     have signs, names to honor a benefactor, etc.?)
Who owns it? Does the person have a chance to invest in the house, or
     are funds used for staff fees, etc.?
Is it close to stores, churches, place of employment, recreation?
Can residents have visitors, snacks whenever they want? Do they have
     sufficient privacy?
Who are the managers? Do they serve as "parents" to residents, while
     they live with other adults?
Do residents participate in planning, cooking, and cleaning? Do they
     have full access to kitchens, laundry facilities, etc. or are these
     confined to "therapy" times?
If you woke up tomorrow morning unable to work or needing
     specialized care, would you be willing to move in?

Pieper also discusses a number of myths that seem to get in the way of clearly and rationally planning for alternative living arrangements. Among these are ideas such as "there will always be those who need institutions" or "people with extensive medical involvement cannot live in normalized settings." Certainly, we can recognize that many adults with disabilities need assistance; but as Pieper puts it, "By what leap of logic do those needs imply that a person requires an institution as we know it?"[7] Often, this "specialized" care is what the parents have been providing for many years. If nonmedical, nonprofessional parents have been able to provide this care and assistance throughout childhood, then it seems reasonable to assume that other adults could also learn to do this with some guidance and training. There are probably very few needs so specialized that they require the services of an entire institution or nursing home.

As each child with a disability reaches adulthood, that individual and his or her family need to think about living arrangements; first in terms of the positive wishes and aspirations of the young person, and secondly in terms of how the disability can be accommodated into those wishes. Planning that *starts* with the disability may neglect many possibilities. The primary focus needs to be on the "normal" needs of the young person for work, recreation, and socialization. When these are clear, the ways in which the disability needs to be considered can be addressed.

Parents will need both concrete information and emotional support as they face the complex questions of adulthood for their children. It is useful to gather information and talk to people in parent groups, groups and coalitions of adults with disabilities, and educational and vocational agencies. Asking questions and collecting information can help parents become familiar with what is available; talking with other parents and adults with disabilities can enable parents to clarify their own feelings and reactions. Decisions made must ultimately "fit" both the young person with the disability and the parents, if they are to have optimal chances of succeeding.

QUESTIONS FOR PARENTS

1. Am I continuing to reassess how much independence my child is capable of, and continuing to move toward greater independence?
2. Is my child continuing to explore interests, hobbies, and activities?
3. Does he or she have opportunities for friendships?
4. Can I talk with my child about his or her hopes for the future?
5. Do I feel that I have reasonably accurate information about my child's intellectual and vocational abilities?
6. Do I know where to look for information about schools, vocational training, and living arrangements?
7. Have I made contact with groups of people with disabilities to explore information and ideas?
8. What kinds of living arrangements are available in my community?
9. What are my own feelings (my hopes, as well as my fears) about my child's "place in the world"?
10. Can my spouse and I share our feelings about our child's future, even though our views may not be the same or we may each be inconsistent ourselves?

REFERENCES

1. Siegel, Ernest, *The Exceptional Child Grows Up*, E. P. Dutton, 1974.
2. Mitchell, Joyce Slayton, *See Me More Clearly: Career and Life Planning for Teens with Physical Disabilities*, Harcourt, Brace Jovanovitch, 1980.
3. Pieper, Betty, *By, For and With . . . Young Adults with Spina Bifida*, Spina Bifida Association of America, 343 S. Dearborn, Chicago, Illinois 60604, 1979.
4. Brewer, Garry D., and Kakalik, James S., *Handicapped Children: Strategies for Improving Services*, McGraw-Hill, 1979.
5. Pendler, Betty, My Daughter is Leaving Home: What Do I Do Now," *The Exceptional Parent*, June 1979.
6. Brown, Sara L., and Dickinson, Martha Ufford in Brown in Brown, Sara L. and Moersch, Martha S., Eds., *Parents on the Team*, University of Michigan Press, 1978.
7. Pieper, Betty, *Beyond the Family and the Institution: Residential Issues for Today*, Spina Bifida Association of America, 343 S. Dearborn, Chicago, Illinois 60604, 1979.

10
ISSUES OF ADOLESCENCE
Sexuality

A discussion of sexuality really belongs at the beginning of a book such as this. Although issues of sex and sexuality are more likely to come out into the open during the teenage years, they have been present all along. Attitudes toward being boys or girls, masculine or feminine, and what it will be like to be "like Mommy" or "like Daddy" have been developing since early childhood. So too have the uses of the physical body to express warmth and affection. Babies and young children share hugs, snuggles, and nose-rubbing with their parents and caretakers; and they know that these are love.

Sex is, as many books on the subject tell us, a difficult subject for parents to address directly and honestly with any child. To do so means that parents must openly face their own sexuality, as well as acknowledge the sexuality of their child. This is often difficult enough for parents of nondisabled children. For parents of children with disabilities, it is often very painful. Disabilities bring in to focus deep attitudes and values concerning physical attractiveness and sexual behavior. They may trigger parents' fears about their children's future when the time comes that parents can no longer care for them and protect them.

Nondisabled children and teenagers, if their parents are unwilling or unable to discuss sexual questions with them, usually have access to friends and peers with whom they can share their curiosity and knowledge. While the information gleaned in this way may be inadequate or incorrect, such sharing at least allows the open acknowledgement of emerging sexual awareness. Many children with disabilities are more limited in these opportunities. Their chances to mingle with a peer group in a variety of activities, including private times for the sharing of "secrets," are often fewer.

Many teenagers and adults with disabilities will say that they have been raised as though they were sexless. They will also say, if they trust the listener, that they most emphatically are *not*. What many of them have faced, sadly, is a vacuum created by the lack of access to sharing with friends, the fears and myths of our society, and their parents' inability to face the difficult issues involved.

These issues are ideally looked at by parents long before their children reach adolescence, while there is time to think and reflect on the questions and on the reactions aroused in parents. Anyone, parent or professional, who is involved with young people making the transition from childhood to adulthood needs to spend some time clarifying his or her own information and attitudes about sex and sexuality. Sex is a value laden area; if we are not clear about what we know and how we feel about it, we are more apt to react according to our own needs rather than the adolescent's. It is my hope that parents of young children will begin the process of thinking about these questions, and of reading and talking with others, so that they may approach their childrens' adolescence with more comfort and confidence.

ISSUES FOR PARENTS

How can a parent of a child with a disability begin to prepare for dealing with questions about the sexuality of that child? The parent can begin early, long before the child is a teenager, to learn and reflect about such areas as:

Recognizing that everyone is sexual. Sexuality is a natural part of the make-up of every person, throughout his or her life.
Recognizing that the messages one conveys to children about values and about being "men" and "women" are often communicated without words in a variety of nonsexual situations.
Being comfortable with one's own sexuality and the choices one makes in expressing it.
Understanding that the child with a disability is as much a sexual being as any other person.
Being approachable to one's children about sex as well as other concerns.
Learning more about sexuality.

THE NATURE OF SEXUALITY

Sexuality is an integral, natural part of the experience of being human. Humans are sexual beings throughout life, from infancy through old age. Since infants and very young children are capable of physical sexual responses, it is important to think of sexuality as more than genital behavior leading to orgasm. Sexuality is more than intercourse; it encompasses a wide variety of physical and emotional pleasures and responses. Feelings and attitudes about one's body, about being male or female, and the ability to experience and to share physical and emotional intimacy are all related to human sexuality.

Parents can thus assume that their children with disabilities are sexual and that they will remain so throughout their lives. The question is not *whether* the child will be sexual; it is *how* his or her sexuality will be acknowledged and expressed.

The importance of this concept cannot be overestimated. Parents, and professionals, who fully accept the sexual component of a child with a disability will interact very differently with that child than will people who find their own or the child's sexuality uncomfortable. Children who sense that sexuality is a topic that arouses anxiety in the adults around them will be less able to obtain the information they need or to come to accept and deal with their own sexual needs and feelings.

It takes courage to look squarely at one's own values about sexuality. It takes even more courage to face the realities of the world with its myths and fears about the sexuality of people who are disabled and to explore the ways of meeting the sexual needs of a disabled individual. When that disabled individual is one's own child, strong feelings about alternative means of sexual expression, masturbation, or the sexual attractiveness to bodies which are "different" may be aroused.

Some of these feelings and attitudes may surprise the parent. Each of us has absorbed throughout our lives, quite unconsciously, a variety of attitudes and values about our physical bodies and sexual expression. It is only when we decide to pull these out of our mental "closets" that we can really see what we have accumulated and stored away. Then it becomes possible to examine our attitudes and values and to decide which of them we wish to keep and which we would like to change.

BODY IMAGE

Acceptance and enjoyment of the sexual component of human nature requires that one be able to accept and enjoy one's physical body. It is difficult to take pleasure in physical bodily responses and to think about sharing those responses with others if one feels that one's body is ugly or unattractive. Parents and professionals who are concerned with the emerging sexuality of adolescents will need to spend some time pondering their own ideas about physical attractiveness. Do they, for example, have idealized images of what kinds and shapes of bodies are sexually attractive? Where do those ideas and images come from?

Is the parent comfortable with his or her own body, even though it does not fit the ideal?

Teenagers with disabilities will need to come to terms with the ways in which their bodies are different from the popularized ideals in magazine and television commercials. Adolescents with disabilities have often had many years of experiences of having their bodies looked at, examined, and treated. Often these repeated examinations are carried out before groups of people in white coats, some of whom the child has not seen before and will not see again. Surgical treatments cause fear, pain, and scars. It is no wonder that many adolescents are accustomed to "divorcing" their physical bodies from their sense of themselves as people, or that they become very adept at ignoring their bodies.

Children and adolescents need to have their bodily integrity respected. Busy clinics, demanding schedules, and inadequate facilities make this difficult. But for the child or teenager, the exposure of the body and the submission to embarrassment and discomfort are not casual matters. Sensitive professionals will quickly realize that it does not take significantly more time to ask the young person's permission for the examination, or to indicate respect by closing doors, pulling curtains, and providing covering for the parts of the body not being examined.

Alert parents can help the shy youngster by avoiding unnecessary exposure and politely reminding professional people about privacy. It helps too for the parent to convey an attitude of acceptance of his or her own body as well as the child's. Parents who can good-naturedly joke about their own imperfections can help the child become comfortable with his or her own. Any attitude on the part of the parent that a part of the child's body is ugly or unacceptable will be quickly picked up, even by a very young child. Parents who find that they have negative reactions to the child's body or appearance may need to explore these feelings with a therapist or counselor so that they will not be transmitted to the child.

HYGIENE

The teenager who has learned to ignore parts of his or her body will have difficulty in caring for those parts. This may be rooted in a desire to deny the parts that do not work or which cause pain. Adolescents with paralyzed legs, for example, often have difficulty in "remembering" to keep the skin of their feet and legs clean and to watch for pressure areas. While this attitude may be natural and understandable, it is a serious barrier both to good hygiene and to the acceptance of the whole body with its limitations and its possibilities. It may be inconceivable to a disabled teenager to think that an "imperfect" part of the body may be a potential source of pleasure to a lover.

Children need to be educated about their bodies in terms they can understand all throughout childhood. They need explanations of how their bodies work, and why operations and treatments have been done. They need to be able to look at and handle their own bodies. They will be better able to do this if the adults who care for them are accepting, open, and matter-of-fact about their bodies.

PRIVACY

Adolescents need private times and private places to explore and become acquainted with their own bodies. This may mean experimenting with clothes, mirrors, and makeup; touching the body; and masturbation. Children with disabilities, like other children, need to know that their bodies are capable of pleasant sexual feelings and that these are natural and expected. The provision of privacy may be difficult for parents who are accustomed to providing assistance with toileting and dressing. Such parents may be in the habit of being with the child in the bedroom or bathroom and may need to think about knocking on the door instead of walking right in.

Privacy may be one thing; but for many parents, masturbation is another. It may be extremely difficult for some parents to accept the idea that masturbation may be a healthy, normal way for their child to learn about and enjoy his or her own sexuality. Here again, the notion that the question is not *whether* the child will be sexual, but rather *how* that sexuality will be handled, may help to put things in perspective. It can certainly be argued that the person who has a means for expressing his or her own sexuality will be less vulnerable to inappropriate or exploitive sexual behavior with others.

It is certainly not suggested that parents feel they must choke down or deny their own feelings. The feelings, values, and attitudes of parents are entitled to as much respect as anyone else's. Parents may, however, want to spend some time thinking about their values and attitudes. Where do they originate from? Are there remnants of old horror stories and myths about masturbation present? What are the facts about masturbation? As in other situations in which parents struggle with strong feelings and conflicts, it can be very helpful to talk these over with other parents in a parents' group or with a professional counselor. Ignoring the questions will not make them disappear. It is far preferable to struggle openly with them than to bury them where they may lead to chronic tension.

PEER GROUP OPPORTUNITIES

Children and adolescents with disabilities may not have the same opportunities as other youngsters to be an integral part of a peer group. This may be the result of a number of factors, only one of which is the disability itself. Children who go to different schools or who ride special buses while their neighbors walk to school do not have the same chances to develop casual friendships or to engage in the sharing of friendly secrets or horseplay on the way to or from school. When visits must be arranged and parents must be involved in the scheduling and transportation, the chances for spontaneous, spur-of-the-moment interactions are greatly reduced.

Adolescence can be a lonely time for young people with disabilities. Other teenagers are consumed during these years with their own needs to be "just like everyone else"; they may have little capacity for the differences of others. The new-found freedom to move about on bicycles or in cars is so exciting that they forget to include the friend who is less mobile. Thus learning about sexual matters and about how to get along with members of the opposite sex is hampered. While this may improve in future years as other teenagers mature and become less self-centered, this is not much comfort to the lonely adolescent.

Teenagers with disabilities may need building of their self-esteem. They may need encouragement from parents to keep involved; to invite friends over, to participate in activities, and to initiate friendships. Parents may find themselves walking a tightrope between encouragement and pushing. Parents may also be tired from years of extra transporting and assistance, and the prospect of keeping pizzas in the house and otherwise making the home into an attractive place for teenagers to congregate may be a dismaying one.

But the opportunity to learn to be comfortable with and to enjoy other people of both sexes is essential. For most people, sexual relationships are only one part of a whole range of relationships that are possible with others. Whether or not the young person with a disability eventually chooses to form sexual relationships, he or she will need to have had some practice in being warm and being friendly with others.

Since young people with disabilities may not have the same opportunities as their peers to share information about sex, it may be especially important for parents to see that their children are educated. Children with disabilities need to know about the sexual functioning of their bodies. Sex education means learning how the body works and about the possibilities of pregnancy. Youngsters who are retarded, no less than others, need to know how babies are conceived and that their own bodies may be capable of pleasurable responses, and that one can make choices about when and with whom to share those responses.

Information about birth control is a vital part of the sex education needs of young people with disabilities. This cannot be taken for granted. Many nondisabled teenage girls become pregnant because they do not know about birth control options or because they have not been encouraged to think in terms of their own personal choices and the implications of those choices. The provision of information about pregnancy and birth control, in the context of each individual's responsibility for his or her own choices, cannot be left to chance. Teenagers with disabilities may not have access to the informal sharing of information among friends; and the statistics on teenage pregnancies tell us that this method of education is woefully inadequate. Young people who are retarded are, more often than we might think, capable of understanding the childrearing would be a very difficult commitment to undertake. These young people deserve to have information that they can understand and the right to participate in decisions about birth control or sterilization.

OPPOSITE-SEX RELATIONSHIPS

Parents who begin to impart information about sex and sexuality early, while their children are young, are ahead of the game. They also will have the chance to confront their own feelings and reactions about the child as a potential sex partner for someone. It may be difficult to think about the child's chances of entering into a loving, sexual relationship. Parents may fear that the child will be lonely and unloved; or they may feel that they themselves could not find a body which is scarred or encumbered with appliances sexually attractive. Such thoughts may arouse strong feelings of guilt or anxiety. The best antidote for these reactions is time; time and using that time to talk with others. Parents who have the courage to talk about these reactions with other parents or with professional counselors will find that with the talking, the unspeakable becomes not only "speakable" but also manageable. There is comfort in the sharing, and with that comfort comes the possibility of looking at sex and sexual expression in different ways.

For what is needed in many situations *is* a totally new perspective on human sexual relationships. If one accepts the premise that all people are sexual and that sexual feelings are not inherently sinful or shameful, then one can be open to considering alternatives. Parents do not need to fear that this means discarding their own values and beliefs. It does mean, however, that it will be necessary to reexamine values about sexual expression in order to determine which of them the parent wishes to retain and which have more flexibility. Many parents will find that sexual behaviors for their children that do not violate values about exploitation, privacy, or the birth of unwanted children may become quite acceptable even though they are different from the parents' own behaviors.

It is, perhaps, the parents who are most loving and physically affectionate with their children who will face the dilemmas most squarely. For if physical expressions of love and closeness — hugging, caressing, and fondling — are important to the parent and child, it may be very painful to think about how, or whether, the child may continue to have these as an adult. Parents feel real pain when they realize that they can no longer be the source of love that was so important in helping the child to grow and flourish. The irony is that "the more attending, caring and loving the family has been, the more the young person knows that his feelings are acceptable and the more he wants to perpetuate those feelings and seek love for himself."[1]

Parents should not be too quick to assume that warm, loving relationships and even marriage are not to be possible for their children. These may well be possible, although perhaps not in exactly the same form as those of the parents. People who are disabled can and do marry; even people with retardation may find satisfactory marriages together. Two retarded people may pool their resources and manage quite well. Janet Mattison, in commenting on a study of previously institutionalized retarded people who were married and living in the community in England, says: "My ultimate conclusion about these former patients of a hospital for the retarded was that, paired, many of them were able to reinforce each other's strengths and established marriages which, in the light of what had happened to them previously, were no more, no less, foolish than many others in the community, and which gave them considerable satisfaction."[2]

Parents who accept the sexuality of their children can begin to think about the responsible expression of that sexuality, and can begin to teach the children about these responsibilities. They can, for example, explain to children who are retarded or who have physical disabilities about their possibilities of becoming parents, and the need to safeguard against the risk of unwanted pregnancies. Parents of children who are retarded may need to begin early to teach children when physical affection is appropriate and when it is not. They may need to explain, for example, why they hug an old friend when she comes to visit and not the door-to-door salesman.[3] Children who are retarded must learn some lessons about the appropriateness of physical closeness if they are to be able to protect themselves from exploitation. It is naive to think that the retarded young person who knows nothing about sex is safe from getting into trouble or being taken advantage of by another. It is the ignorant young person who is most vulnerable to inappropriate behavior or to the advances of unscrupulous others. In the words of John W. Money, "The mentally retarded also have to develop their own moral standards, and we have to help them to do so."[4]

The dilemma of the parents or other caretakers of persons with a greater degree of retardation, when it comes to making decisions about the retarded persons' fertility, is a complex and difficult one. Even experts have differences of opinion as to when measures such as sterilization may be appropriate — for example, when the retarded person will not be able to care for a child. Historically, (and even not so historically), sterilization has been considered as an option not so much for the benefit of the retarded person but to assuage the fears of society that unbridled sexuality would be rampant if unsterilized retarded people were to be in the community. If sterilization is to be considered, the person who is retarded must be involved actively in the decision and every care must be taken to safeguard his or her rights. As Robert Burt says, "This special vulnerability of mental retardates [to fears of unabated sexual appetites] means that, as a group, they warrant particular protection, most notably against the operation of legislation aimed at their sexual and childrearing behavior."[5]

This means that the needs of the individual retarded young person, along with those of any potential children, need to be the primary focus of discussions relating to decisions about contraceptive methods or sterilization. Decisions applied to "the retarded" as a group, or which are based primarily on the fears of the community, are profoundly unjust. Sterilization as an option must be approached with particular caution. Sterilization techniques, today, are not reliably reversible; thus such decisions must be considered to be permanent. Some retarded persons *will* be able to support themselves and care for children, and this possibility should not be closed off too quickly.

Parents who are grappling with the questions of sexuality and birth control will need to learn more about birth control methods. Oral contraceptives, because they require daily attention, may not be an ideal choice for the retarded young woman. An intrauterine device (IUD) might offer less worrisome protection. For men, the condom, with proper instruction in its use, probably still represents the best choice.

Other dilemmas are faced by parents whose teenage or young adult children are physically disabled. If the disability severely limits the young person's ability to move about or to tend to his or her own body, sexual expression may mean that help is required. In its simpler forms, this need for help may mean that the parents are involved in transporting their children on dates and wrestling with questions about providing privacy for more intimate conversations and closeness for their young adult and another. In some cases, however, the person's movement may be restricted enough to actually require some assistance in arranging for masturbation or other sexual activity. For many parents, the difference between knowing that sexual activity is taking place and actually helping to make that activity possible is very large indeed. This issue may be faced not only by parents but also by professionals or other caretakers who are in a position to give or to withhold the help that the young person needs. Whether or not that help can be freely given, the disabled young person deserves to have the question thought about and to have his or her sexual needs taken into account. Discrepancies between the parent's own standards and the child's special circumstances will need to be examined and worked through.

THE YOUNG PERSON'S NEED FOR INFORMATION

Young people with disabilities, as much as their nondisabled peers, need information on sexuality in general and on their own particular situation. This is just as true for young people who are retarded as it is for those with physical disabilities. Sol Gordon has summed up the basic rights of retarded young people in the area of sexuality as follows: (Although this was written in reference to institutions, the basic ideas expressed here are appropriate to all concerned with the retarded.)

1. People with special needs, as all people, should have easy access to information on sexuality and birth control.
2. Masturbation is a normal expression of sex no matter how frequently it is done and at what age. It becomes a compulsive, punitive, self-destructive behavior largely as a result of guilt, suppression and punishment.
3. All direct sexual behavior involving the genitals should be in privacy. (Recognizing that institutions and hospitals for the retarded . . . are not built or developed to ensure privacy, the definition of what constitutes privacy in an institution must be very liberal — bathrooms, one's own bed, the bushes, basements are private domains.)
4. Anytime a physically mature girl and a boy have sexual relations, they risk pregnancy.
5. Unless they are clear about wanting a baby and the responsibility that goes with child-rearing, both the male and female should use birth control. (Staff should not condition girls of any age to believe that every woman wants and must have babies in order to be 'normal.') Birth control services and genetic counseling should be available to all disabled adults.

6. Until you are, say, 18, society feels you should not have intercourse. After this, you decide for yourself — providing you use birth control.
7. Adults should not be permitted to use children sexually.
8. In the final analysis, sexual behavior between consenting adults (regardless of mental age) and whether it is homo or hetero, should be no one else's business — providing there is little risk of bringing an unwanted child into this world.[3]

It is only with accurate information and the opportunity to come to grips with their own sexuality that young people with disabilities will be able to experience that sexuality in ways that are not harmful to themselves or to others. Obviously, this information must be geared to individual person's knowledge, experience, and vocabulary. It will do no good to talk about "intercourse" or "masturbation" to a young retarded person who does not comprehend what those words mean.

Young adults with physical disabilities will, as they begin to contemplate how they will be able to relate to other people sexually, need some very specific information in addition to the general facts about sex and childbearing. They will need to know how their own bodies work in relation to sex and to possible parenthood. Girls with spina bifida, for example, may assume that because they have difficulty with bladder functioning, they are also unable to become pregnant. This is an incorrect and obviously dangerous assumption. Boys will need to know about how and under what conditions they might expect to have erections. Both sexes will need to have access to accurate information about their physical capabilities. Parents will not have all the answers to these questions. What they may be able to do is to steer the young person to professionals who are qualified to answer them and to other written materials (see in Appendix B).

More information is becoming available in written form about the struggle to be seen as a complete person even with a disability. Young adults can benefit from reading about, for example, how to look "sexy" in a wheelchair or by joining discussion groups of other young adults to talk about common experiences. Parents will know they have succeeded when their adult children can deal with their sexuality in ways that are satisfying and not harmful to themselves or others. Much of the groundwork for this success can be laid during childhood.

QUESTIONS FOR PARENTS

1. Am I comfortable with my own sexuality and its place in my life?
2. Can I explore the roots of my values about sex and sexual expression?

3. Do I still carry around some myths about sexuality that are no longer useful to me?
4. Can I help my child to feel comfortable about his or her own body?
5. Can I imagine my child having sexual feelings and responses?
6. If I know that my child has masturbated, is it upsetting to me?
7. What are my wishes for my child as an adult, in terms of having warm and intimate relationships?
8. What are my fears about that?
9. Do I know where I can get more information for myself or for my child in the area of sexuality?

REFERENCES

1. Dickinson, Martha Ufford and Brown, Sara L., in *Parents on the Team*, University of Michigan Press, 1978.
2. Mattison, Janet, Marriage and Mental Handicap, in de La Cruz, Felix F. and La Veck, Gerald D., Eds., *Human Sexuality and the Mentally Retarded*, Brunner-Mazel, 1973.
3. Gordon, Sol, *Sexual Rights for the People . . . Who Happen to be Handicapped*, Syracuse, Center on Human Policy, 1974.
4. Money, John W., Some Thoughts on Sexual Taboos and the Rights of the Retarded, in de La Cruz, Felix F. and La Veck, Gerald D., Eds., *Human Sexuality and the Mentally Retarded*, Brunner-Mazel, 1973.
5. Burt, Robert A., Legal Restrictions on Sexual and Familial Relations of Mental Retardates — Old Laws, New Guises, in de La Cruz, Felix F. and La Veck, Gerald D., Eds., *Human Sexuality and the Mentally Retarded*, Brunner-Mazel, 1973.

11
LEARNING TO BE AN ADVOCATE

"An advocate!" many people will exclaim, "What an awesome prospect for me." The word advocacy may evoke images of picket lines, sit-ins, or Carrie Nation charging into saloons in her battle against the evils of alcohol. But advocacy need not automatically mean the use of aggressive or confrontational tactics. Advocacy, in its most general sense, means looking out for and speaking on behalf of the interests of someone else. To be an advocate, one must represent the needs and rights of another, without conflicts of interest or divided loyalties.

Responsible advocacy for the needs of people with disabilities encompasses many areas. It includes acquiring knowledge about what the needs of persons with disabilities are; learning about the services; building relationships and increasing communication with the providers of services and the public; suggesting alternative solutions to problems; and educating people about disabilities and the gaps that exist in services and opportunities. There is plenty of room in the field of advocacy for those who are more comfortable working behind the scenes in collecting information or planning strategy.

Is advocacy still necessary in today's world? For many parents, the answer to this question is an emphatic "Yes!" These are the families who are confronted with a rude shock when they are ready to turn their attention from their own internal adjustment and management of the disability to the community and world about them. Families may have struggled mightily to adapt to a child's disability and to find a new balance in their lives as families. They have incorporated the disability into the joys and pains of living and are ready to go on with the business of their lives.

The shock is the awareness that the rest of our society does not see disabilities the way that parents do. The attitudes of parents have changed and become different, but society's have not. Our society continues to place a high premium on youth, beauty, slimness, and intelligence. People tend to be uncomfortable with wheelchairs, crutches, hearing aids, or obvious "differences" in appearance or mannerisms. Parents discover that other people cannot look as easily beyond the trappings of the disability as parents can.

The observant parent will notice that our society may be quick to espouse equal opportunities for people with disabilities in the abstract, but many, many problems arise in specific cases. Schools, public buildings, and transportation systems are not designed for wheelchairs or Braille markings. Needed programs may be "offered" only after prolonged battles. Each group home established must survive heated and prolonged resistance from the neighborhood it is in. Many are lost in these battles for each that survives to be built. Opportunities for housing, recreation, and work for those over age 18 with disabilities who require some assistance are pitifully inadequate.

Many inconsistencies exist in the distribution of services and educational programs throughout the country as well as sources of information about what services are available, how to locate appropriate services, or even in the ways to learn about what the alternatives are.[1] Inequities and inconsistencies exist in the area of financial aid, too. Many states will exclude from assistance those families who earn enough to support and care for themselves under usual circumstances but who cannot afford to pay for the specialized treatment and care a child may require. However, if the family "gives up" and places the child in foster care, the child will have not only her extra care paid for but also her basic expenses for food and clothing. The state thus pays more than it would to provide assistance to the natural family. However, with help and support, more natural families could keep their children.

Other families, whose children are receiving needed services in treatment, education, and transportation, may be more dubious about the need for advocacy. "We can relax now," they say, "our children have the services they need." Certainly, significant progress *has* been made in the last few decades. But what these parents sometimes neglect to consider is the fact that although needed services may be available and working well while the child is still a child, the situation will probably change drastically when that child becomes an adult. Suddenly, at age 18 or 21, opportunities for education for the retarded, for example, are no longer automatically available. Places where people with disabilities can live away from home independently but with some assistance are few and far between.

Parents whose children are or are about to become adults already know this. Parents of younger children may prefer not to think ahead to what kinds of options will be available or what kind of life the child will have; but if they wait, it may be too late. It is already too late for many adults with disabilities.

It is prudent to have an alert advocacy effort "in place" even when things are going well, because problems can and do arise. Budget difficulties, personnel changes, or changing emphases may threaten existing services. When this happens, the people who are affected need to be able to react. If the advocacy system is in place and ready, this reaction can be prompt. If, however, it is necessary to start over again by contacting people, collecting information, and setting up a system of committees and action, much valuable time will be lost. The reaction of the people affected by proposed changes will be much less effective, and may be too late.

Thus advocacy is still very much needed in today's world. Gaps in services still exist. Many people do not have adequate access to the most appropriate services or even to information about those services. Attitudinal barriers are slow to change; the passage of laws legitimizes the bases for insisting on equal rights and opportunities, but it cannot do a great deal to change deep-seated attitudes and prejudices. Patient and persistent educational programs are needed. Often the people responsible for implementing a new law do not fully understand the meaning or the spirit of that law. This has led to wheelchair-sized bathrooms located in corners where wheelchairs cannot turn around and curb ramps being installed around an existing telephone pole, leaving the pole in the center of the ramp.

The sands of public opinion and public pressure shift frequently. Programs seen as desirable one year may come under attack the next when budget cuts are threatened. The pressures of today's national economic situation threaten not only needed new programs but also the hard-won gains already achieved. An advocacy effort that continually monitors services, even in good times, will be available to lobby in defense of endangered services.

WHO SHALL ADVOCATE?

The advocacy we are speaking of is one that incorporates awareness of the needs and rights of the disabled as a group into action designed to meet those needs and rights. This is the advocacy carried out by voluntary groups and organizations as well as concerned individuals. Advocates who are designated to represent specific individuals with disabilities at hearings or other sessions where decisions are made regarding that disabled individual will need more information and training than this chapter can provide.

regarding that disabled individual will need more information and training than this chapter can provide.

The realm of advocacy has room for all who are interested in securing equal opportunities for people with disabilities. Obviously, people with disabilities, and their families, have intimate knowledge of the needs and problems as well as a strong vested interest in the availability of services. But there are many practical reasons for incorporating a wide base of support into the advocacy effort. There is a danger that consumers may be "tuned out" by the public, legislatures, or service providers simply because their interests are so obviously personal. The inclusion of professionals, service providers, legislators, clergy, and a variety of community leaders helps to insure that the message will be listened to.

Many parents struggle with the idea of becoming an advocate. The prospect seems difficult, and the need for it unfair. "We have enough to do in being parents, and citizens, and trying to lead our own lives," they say. And they are right. But it is also true that no one else can bring to the arena of debate the unique perspective of the parent or the person who actually "owns" the disability. Others who advocate are likely to have other loyalties in addition to their commitment to the disabled. They are not faced with living, day by day, with the results of decisions in the same way that persons with disabilities and their families are.

Parents who are involved in lobbying or public education on a local level may be uncomfortable in seeming to be asking for help for their own child. Somehow, it seems a bit like asking for favors, or for "charity." But there is a very important difference between asking for charity or special concessions and asking for a fair shake. No parent need feel apologetic about speaking out on behalf of equal opportunities for all persons with disabilities. It is the people who understand what disabilities and inadequate services mean in human terms who are most likely to support efforts for change. The voice of the parent, or the person with the disability, is a unique source of that human dimension.

Parents or others who are interested in advocacy may fear that this is a very lonely venture. This is not necessarily so. If a parent, a professional, or a person with a disability recognizes a need or an inequity, the chances are good that this has been noticed by others, or that other individuals and groups would be receptive to sharing in the effort. Many organizations of people with disabilities and parents currently exist. These groups have usually been dealing with issues and problems related to the need the parent or individual sees, if not the specific manifestation of that problem. The individual who would like to begin advocating can attend meetings of parent groups or other organizations concerned with disabilities. Listening, asking questions, and sharing information can reveal the potential for increased effectiveness which can result from pooling efforts and information. Statements made by a group or an organization may carry more weight than those made by individuals; and the individual can benefit from the support and comfort that comes from sharing the battles.

Groups and organizations concerned with disabilities are not only sources of potential allies. Community, civic, and church groups may also be interested once they are informed about the problems. It takes a certain amount of groundwork to plan an approach for bringing an issue to an organization's attention. If it is a community group, it may be necessary to offer to speak or present a program on disabilities or the needs that exist. Many such groups simply do not realize the inequities confronted by people with disabilities. Often, increased understanding brings a desire to help. Parent or disability groups that can provide speakers to go out into the community can increase public consciousness and awareness as well as recruit volunteers.

If one wishes to facilitate formal action on the part of the organization in question, it is usually necessary to learn something about how the group operates. Who, for example, sets the agenda for meetings? Does the group have a committee that should be contacted first? Who is in charge of the appropriate committee? Learning about these things in advance helps to avoid the frustration of failing because the "right" people were not contacted or because the proposal did not mesh with the way the group functions.

Parents or others who think about advocacy as something that they ought or would like to do often fear that they lack the necessary skills. They may envision advocacy primarily in terms of eloquent public speaking. But effective advocacy encompasses many of the skills and abilities that we use in everyday life. When a parent requests a conference with a teacher because a "normal" child is being bullied on the playground, or when a person returns a defective product to a store and requests a refund, they are using advocacy skills. The abilities that enable us to look at a situation and see what is missing, to suggest alternative solutions, and to talk to others about what we need are all useful advocacy skills. There is no magic in advocacy.

But parents may ask, does this mean that we must bear the brunt of the burden? Can't the professional people who provide the services do the advocating? Of course they can advocate, often very effectively. There are many caring, concerned people in the "system" who do a great deal to further the cause of equal opportunities for the disabled. But even well-meaning, caring people may disagree about what is "best" in a given situation. People in the system, even those with the best of intentions, do have some limitations. Some loyalty is bound to exist to the agency or institution paying one's salary.

In very practical terms, there may be limits as to how far one can go in confronting and challenging one's own agency without risking severe displeasure or even possible loss of the job itself. Consumers, on the other hand, do not have to face these constraints. They are free to speak publicly about their criticisms and to mobilize support for change. Many concerned professionals know this and will seek out, "off the record," voluntary groups of consumers with whom to share their perceptions and dilemmas. These professionals recognize that some situations call for the kind of public pressure that they, in their official positions, cannot provide.

The most successful advocacy efforts are usually those with as wide a base of support as possible. Different groups of people will pay attention to different "experts" for different problems. Professionals, statisticians, legislators, and community leaders can be as vital to success as the consumer.

STRATEGIES OF ADVOCACY

In the following pages, we will be discussing approaches to advocacy. The discussion will begin with the more general or philosophical issues of advocacy. Although some more specific areas will be addressed, this chapter is not, basically, a "how-to" manual. Others of these have been written, and the reader will find some of these references in Appendix B, Advocacy.

This discussion assumes that advocacy is an effort to make something *different*. Presumably, the person who advocates is aware of a situation that is felt to be unsatisfactory, and seeks to make a change to improve that situation. It is essential, however, to avoid the trap of focusing first and only on the solution, or on ways to "fix" the undesirable situation. Our frustration and impatience often lead us directly into this trap. But when we jump directly to solutions, we are in real danger of overlooking many factors that may result in a worsening rather than an improving of the situation. In the 1960s, a genuine wish to improve the treatment of the chronically mentally ill led to an enthusiastic push for emptying isolated state mental hospitals and returning people to their home communities. But the implications of this well-intentioned effort, in terms of the availability of services in the communities, the funding needed for those services, and the willingness of the communities to accept the chronically mentally ill, were not sufficiently addressed. The sad result is that many of these people are actually worse off than before.

PHILOSOPHICAL UNDERPINNINGS OF ACTION

The quest for solutions can distract from the consideration of wider issues of social climate and attitude. This is particularly true in advo- cating for a group that has historically been perceived as "disadvan- taged" or "in need of charity." People who are to serve as advocates need to search their own attitudes and examine the attitudes they wish to foster. The ends, whether increased services or financial support, can obscure the wider implications of the means. With regard to people with disabilities, this can be boiled down to the question: Is the intent to foster dignity and equality of opportunity, or to ask for "help" in the form of charity?

There is no question that poster children and telethons have en- joyed remarkable success in stimulating the public to contribute to organizations for the disabled. But to what instincts do these ap- proaches appeal? Basically, they aim to make the public uncomfor- table or guilty enough to take the time to write a check or make a pledge. The implication is that that is all that is being asked, and all that needs to be done. When we have experienced sufficient pity, guilt or fear to make a pledge, we can then relax in the knowledge that we have done what we were asked to do.

But what about what we were *not* asked to do? Where is the information about the needs of those children in wheelchairs for dignity, for respect, and for equal access to opportunities for educa- tion and living? Where is the message that adults with disabilities seek not pity but a fair chance to participate in, and contribute to, all aspects of life?

If one has an interest in changing attitudes as well as providing opportunities, then the message chosen and the tactics used do become critical. If we appeal to pity, we encourage an attitude of condescen- sion. Such an appeal does not challenge the basic attitude that we are acting "for" a group of people who are less fortunate than we. If, however, we are operating from a premise that all people are entitled to rights and opportunities regardless of whether or not they are dis- abled, then we will choose appeals to dignity, respect, and fair play. We will then emphasize abilities, not disabilities.

It is important to recognize, however, that emphasizing abilities, or those people who succeed even though they have disabilities, may not achieve very much in the way of basic attitude change. The stigma of handicap is both deep and pervasive. People with disabilities who challenge the stereotypes by succeeding are seen as exceptions to the rule.[2] The basic perception of the disabled as "handicapped" and different remains unchanged.

We need to broaden our thinking beyond the immediate problem at hand and to question the assumptions under which we, and others, operate. Sometimes, it is necessary to ask *why* a question is being raised instead of immediately launching into a debate on it. For example, the issue of whether or not to provide surgical treatment for newborns with some serious birth defects is one that arises not infrequently. It is helpful in such instances to ask why we are considering such an option in these cases. Why, for example, is it "acceptable" to consider withholding treatment from a newborn, but not from a 6-year old who has been hit by a car?

A related trap is that of thinking that what exists is what is needed. If people with disabilities are in special programs or special group homes, we may assume that more of them are needed. Perhaps so; but maybe not. Before leaping into the fray we need to expand our thinking to include larger questions of "Why?" and "Why not?" Do we assume that existing programs and alternatives represent the entire range of solutions? We need to be more creative in our thinking before entering into action.

Finally, a word of caution. Any effort at advocacy carries with it some implication that the advocate does in fact know what is "best" for the person or people being advocated for. Any able-bodied person who speaks on behalf of children or adults with disabilities is still a nondisabled person who is trying to understand the position and needs of people with disabilities. It is imperative that this understanding be somewhat tentative; and that the advocate listen carefully to others who are disabled. As Douglas Biklen put it, "If we think we know what is best for others, we must learn to let others speak for themselves."[3] Trying to *know* what is best for others is risky at best. Effective advocates must continue the process of testing and questioning their assumptions about other people's needs.

Recent years have seen an increase in advocacy efforts by people with disabilities. Organizations of disabled adults have formed, and they have begun to speak publicly about the problems they face and the need for action. The nondisabled advocate, whether parent, professional, or concerned citizen, needs to be clear in his or her own mind that the people who really know about what life is like for the disabled are the people who have the disabilities. While those of us who do not actually have disabilities at this time in our lives can be effective in helping to support social programs and social change, we cannot and should not seek to usurp the primary role that rightfully belongs to those others.

Advocacy activities can be a powerfully positive force in the lives of young people and adults with disabilities. Such activities can be an opportunity to take positive and constructive action instead of feeling helpless and passive. This does not mean that every young person needs to feel that he or she "should" be involved in advocacy. But those who do wish to make a contribution to social change often find that there are personal benefits as well. The opportunity to join forces and share with others and the increased self-confidence which comes from such participation can be valuable fringe benefits.

DEVELOPING AN AWARENESS OF HOW THINGS HAPPEN

Before launching into a plan of action, it is wise to step back first and survey the general climate. How are decisions made in the area that you are interested in? Who are the key people involved in that process? What are the critical points in the process of decision-making? If you are interested in legislative change, for example, then it is necessary to know at least the rudiments of the legislative process. Information about the people who will be likely to support or oppose a bill and what committees that bill must pass through are key elements in planning action.

Good preparation requires a sense of the interrelatedness of social structure and institutions. If a change is made in one area, how will it affect other areas? Problems often arise because not enough attention has been given to the impact of a change. In many cases, for example, "mainstreaming" children with disabilities into regular classrooms was supported and encouraged without addressing adequately the needs and concerns of teachers or the fears of other parents. Paving the way by listening to and dealing with the concerns of people involved, however irrational we may think them to be at first glance, may be necessary.

We live in a complex world of different people with different needs, attitudes, and motivations. These differences result in currents of forces that push and pull in different directions. In thinking about how to bring about change, we need to recognize that some forces operate to encourage the change we have in mind. These are, in Lewin's words, the "driving forces."[4] Others, the "restraining forces" act to discourage or hold back change. Both need to be identified and considered in planning strategy. Increasing the driving forces may seem easiest and most natural. We are most at home with those who think as we do and want what we want. But if the restraining forces are ignored, they too may react and band together in resistance and hostility. Anticipating where resistance is likely to be encountered and acting, in advance, to decrease that resistance will increase the chances of success.

USING A PROBLEM-SOLVING APPROACH

Most people are stimulated to become active in seeking social change
when they are upset: when they are angry or frustrated with the situation
as they see it. To be sure, such emotion is necessary to a sustained
commitment to advocacy efforts. But careful planning and
thoughtful analysis are also needed. The basic problem-solving model
is one that can be used to help channel this emotional energy in the
most constructive way. The model has five steps, and each is important.

1. The first step is to define the problem. At first glance, this
may seem so obvious as to be laughable. "That's easy," says parent A,
"the problem is that my child is not receiving the services she needs at
school." "Well," says parent B, "the problem is that there is not
enough money for the program." "No," says parent C, "the real problem
is that the teachers and administrators do not understand the
need." "You're both wrong," says parent D, "the problem is that the
other parents don't want more special programs in the school." If
parents E, F, and G are present, they will probably offer three more
definitions of the problem. If the problem is not clearly and thoughtfully
defined, some perfectly good solutions may fail because they are
aimed at the wrong problem. In the early stages of problem definition,
all facets of the problem need to be kept in mind. In the example
above, all four parents might be right. If that is the case, then a single
approach will probably not accomplish very much. Multiple problems
demand multiple solutions.

2. The second step is to generate possible solutions. This is best
done in a brain-storming session. Each person present may call out
possible solutions which are then recorded. No effort is made to
evaluate or judge the idea, no matter how impractical or zany it may
sound. There will be plenty of time later to refine or discard suggestions.
Sometimes, the germ of an innovative and successful approach
is found in someone's "crazy" idea. It may well be that one of the
problems in the slowness of progress of opportunities for those who
are disabled is our tendency to continue in the same stale approaches.
New approaches, even "surprises," may be needed. Betty Pieper, for
example, describes an idea for a poster with a child with a kitten in
her lap sitting in a wheelchair, bearing the words "Why are Grown
Men (or the School Board) Afraid of this Child?"[5] But it is not
necessary to reinvent the wheel. Read about how others have tried to
solve problems, and learn from their successes and failures.

3. Once all possible solutions have been generated, the next step
is to evaluate and assess each solution proposed. Here, it is time to
consider what resources are available to help in the effort. What are
the advantages of each solution? What are the costs, or disadvantages?

The range of choices may extend all the way from public education and lobbying to picketing and sit-ins. An effort should be made to consider the overall system in which the problem exists. What parts of the system will the solution affect? If sit-ins and pickets are used, for example, will this generate more publicity? Will it cost the support of some people who disapprove of these tactics? If public education is a solution, what other groups can be asked to help in the effort?

4. The fourth step is to put into effect the designated solution. Here careful definition and follow-through are necessary. It is not enough to adjourn a meeting with a decision of, "We will have a campaign of public education about disabilities." Who will carry out such a campaign? When? What part of the public is meant? How will they be educated: by leaflets, speakers, posters, or what? What will the message say? Unless a specific mechanism is established that clearly specifies who is responsible and when, good intentions are apt to go nowhere.

5. The fifth step is often neglected: we tend to put programs and efforts in motion and to continue on to the next problem without looking back to evaluate what has been achieved. That is how we find programs still in place because "we've always done it that way." It is necessary to look carefully at the solution and its effects to see if it is working. If it is not, it can be altered or discarded. New problems that may be evident can be approached with the same five steps used on the original problem.

DEALING WITH BUREAUCRACIES

The word "bureaucracy" conjures up images of monolithic power, unfeeling immobility, and mazes of rules and regulations. Yet many of the agencies and institutions families and parents come into contact with are bureaucracies. Schools, hospitals, and social service agencies are all bureaucratic organizations. If these negative images remain unchanged, the family will be stuck in a feeling of frustration and helplessness. For the family to have a reasonable chance of getting what it needs from "the system," it must develop some ways of learning about and dealing with that system.

People who feel helpless in their frustration are not likely to get their problems solved. It is necessary for parents to develop some strategies for dealing with bureaucracies and a sense that some things can be done. The first strategy is to remember that agencies and bureaucracies are created to meet the needs of people. "To move bureaucracies you must constantly bear in mind that bureaucrats are public servants; that they are paid by you to provide services for you and your child; that you are the master, they are the servants — not

the other way around."[6] Agencies are the tools by which things get
done; if things are not being done, then people need to look for other
ways to get the tools to work better.

The second strategy for dealing with bureaucracies is to change
them from being impersonal, faceless institutions into more manageable
groups of individual people. It is necessary to meet the actual people
who work in the bureaucracy and to see them, or at least some of them,
as real human beings. While it is necessary to think carefully about how
one wishes to present one's case, it is also necessary to find out something about how the bureaucracy works and who the key people are
in the process. Somewhere in that bureaucratic maze there are likely
to be people whom one can like and respect, and who will help in
explaining the system and planning for strategy. It is worthwhile to
search for these people. In a clinic or hospital, this may be a clinic
coordinator, a social worker, a physician, or some other professional.
In a public school system it may be an administrator, a principal, or
a teacher. Finding a person within the bureaucracy who listens with
understanding and respect does a great deal to eliminate the "them
against us" feeling. It can also provide very useful clues as to how to
proceed so as to be most effective.

The third strategy when preparing to influence a bureaucracy is
to mobilize and broaden the base of support for the proposed change.
If the need is real and the cause is just, then other individuals and
groups are likely to share that need or the belief in the fairness of the
solution. Parents need to look actively for other parents, adults with
disabilities, and groups (both disabled and nondisabled community
groups) to support the effort for change. The "master" of the tools
of bureaucracies and social agencies is more powerful when it represents
a wider range of the citizenry. There is more clout with larger numbers.

It is well to prepare carefully for meetings with representatives
of an agency or institution. The message one wants to convey needs
to be thought through so that it can be presented calmly, clearly,
and convincingly. If one wishes to be listened to with attention and
respect, then one must also be prepared to extend the same to the
other people at the meeting.

But attention and respect do not mean that one must be satisfied
with glib or evasive answers. Most people who have been involved in
struggles for change have heard the following statements, or variations
of them, many times:

"There is simply not enough money"
"You'll have to take away from someone else's program to get what
    you want"
"We've made a lot of progress in this area"

"We're doing as much as we can"
"We'll look into it for you"

There is usually some truth in all of these statements. Advocates should, of course, not hesitate to give credit for efforts that have been made. But it is necessary to stick with the basic premises one has about the needs that exist and the issues of fairness. Of course there is not enough money to do everything. There is even less now than there was 20 years ago. But our society constantly makes choices and sets priorities on what to fund. If certain programs for the disabled did not exist before and "we can't afford to add them now," then people with disabilities are being penalized for what didn't exist before. Maybe it *is* time to question priorities for spending, but to include, for example in education, items like gyms and football uniforms in the list of priorities to be considered.

If, in discussions with people in the bureuacracy, one gets to "We'll look into it," it is time to get more specific. Who will look into it? When will they report back with their findings? Who will they report back to? When will this information be available? Careful follow-through on an issue is every bit as important as careful researching of the needs and careful presentation of the facts. Many good ideas and programs are lost because of inadequate follow-through or inadequate funding support once the concept has been agreed upon.

DEALING WITH PEOPLE

Any effort to advocate means persuading and convincing people. Regardless of whether it is the public, a School Board, an administrator, or a legislature, individual people must hear the message and be persuaded if the effort is to be successful. All of the communication abilities, or "people skills," the advocate has will be useful. The would-be advocate must learn to pay attention to the individuals involved. Tact and diplomacy are especially essential when one feels angry and frustrated. The amenities should be observed even if when the effort to "win someone over" has failed. Guests at meetings, for example, should be greeted courteously and thanked for attending. It is wise to assume when one is trying to persuade that the other person is a human being who might be more receptive at another time, or with another approach. There won't *be* another time if that person becomes too angered or alienated.

Listening is a key to persuading. Often we are so busy planning our rebuttal or our next argument that we do not really hear what the other is saying. Listening carefully means suspending judgement long enough really to hear both the words and the tone of voice of the other. It may help us to arrive at some understanding of why the other person feels as he or she does. This is especially important in areas relating to disabilities, where unspoken attitudes and prejudices may exist. Once we have a better understanding, we are in a better position to plan an approach.

The advocate needs to be clear on the difference between assertion and aggression. Using tact does not mean being wishy-washy or backing down too readily. Assertion is standing firm in relation to oneself or one's cause. Aggression is attacking others. The assertive advocate can remain firm and not take "no" for an answer. "I'm sorry, but I just don't see that those are sufficient reasons for discontinuing this program. The needs still exist, and I will continue to work to save the program," might be an assertive response.

Confidence and the ability to stand firm are greatly enhanced if the advocate is sure of his or her facts. This means collecting information and reviewing it until it is thoroughly familiar. It is helpful to practice presenting the case. The advocate can think up, either alone or in a group, the most awkward or challenging questions that could be asked, and practice responding to them. Even with such practice, however, there are likely to be times when the advocate is caught by questions for which he or she does not have an answer. In such situations, it is wisest to say truthfully, "I don't have that information right now — but I'll be glad to try to find it and get back to you."

Confident advocates recognize the expertise of others, but they do not minimize their own. Advocates may not have degrees in "advocacy" or "voluntary associations," but their knowledge and expertise may be just as valid as a degree in another field. An awareness of the value and solidity of this knowledge is good protection against being intimidated by the degrees or the titles of others.

Successful advocates have an awareness of their own anger. Anger is often a positive force that mobilizes people to become active and to work for change. Anger needs to be admitted and recognized, but not allowed to poison the effort or to blind the advocate to the reactions of others. The advocate may wish to share that anger within the safety of the planning group or committee. For example, he or she might say, "I feel enraged by this decision, but I don't want my rage to sabotage my presentation." This does not mean that anger should never be shown in public; but ideally the advocate should control and utilize its appearance rather than be carried away by it.

DEALING WITH LEGISLATURES

It is necessary from time to time to deal with legislatures. Some problems that families face are not "private" problems; they are reflections of larger social probelms and must be dealt with on that level. The same kinds of strategies and approaches we have considered before apply to dealing with legislatures. One needs some sense of how the process works; how a change in laws is made and what the key decision points are along the way. One also needs to identify the individual people who are in those key positions and to make personal contact with them.

Here it is especially important to seek out and join forces with other groups who support the cause. The larger the constituency supporting a change, the more likely its position will be taken seriously. In addition, other groups and individuals may have valuable experience and contacts to contribute to the effort. Cooperation can avoid much duplication of effort. Instead of a number of groups simultaneously trying to follow a bill's progress, for example, one person or one committee can keep abreast of legislative activities. Then, when critical hearings or meetings are scheduled, that person can notify each group which can then alert its own members to appear in support of a bill.

The following additional suggestions are from the Spina Bifida Association of Delaware Valley (Pennsylvania).

Some legislators think the needs of the handicapped are a bottomless pit. This may be an exaggeration of the facts, but the ability to represent a cause before a legislative body can be improved with the proper techniques.

1. Put yourself in your legislator's shoes. He or she is very busy with a number of issues. When you communicate, keep your story short and present data to the office for study.
2. Whenever possible, check through and seek the advice of the legislator's chief staff person. Whenever written material is left, be sure it is concise and accurate. Acknowledge there is another side to the issue, so the staff person can attempt to reconcile positions. Remember, politics is the art of compromise.
3. Consult with groups that support your position in advance to eliminate differences. You can speed up your cause by securing the consensus in writing to save time and get on with the business of converting the issue into action.
4. Never use loaded data. Be honest and straightforward. If the proposal is going to cost more money, say so. Outline what benefits or disadvantages can arise from the issue. If there are true savings to be realized, point them out in your position paper.
5. Make a personal visit. When you secure your legislator's time ask how many may and should attend. Advise your legislator of meaningful facts and, if it appears a particular point is unfamiliar, offer to help the person gain more knowledge.

Personal appearances and contacts are not the only way to communicate with legislators. Most legislators are sensitive to grass-roots opinions and will pay attention to thoughtful, sincere letters. Letters should be courteous and legible; they also should be addressed properly. Comments put in the writer's own words are generally more effective than form letters. Letters should be brief and to the point. It is best if they refer specifically to the bill's number and title, and if they are received early in the session that is to consider the bill. It is also important to remember to write when the legislator does something that is approved of; most legislators get a lot more criticism than they do praise.

Social change is not easy to achieve. It is quite possible to follow all of the advice in this chapter and still fail. This is intended to be a guide, to help in transforming huge, overwhelming situations and problems into problems with manageable pieces. Success is often achieved in very small steps. Even failure may help to pave the way for greater success on the next try.

QUESTIONS FOR PARENTS

1. Am I aware of what services are provided in my community?
2. Do I know where the unmet needs are?
3. Am I familiar with the people and organizations in my community who are concerned with those needs?
4. Do I know where to turn if I experience problems?
5. Do I have a sense of where the decision points (in agencies, in the community, or in the state legislature) are located?
6. Do I have a clear idea of the "spirit" of services and opportunities that I seek?
7. Do I keep that idea in mind when weighing alternative solutions or strategies?
8. Am I confident about the difference between "charity" and "equal opportunities"?
9. Do I underestimate my own abilities: to collect information, to organize, to plan, or to speak to individuals or groups?

REFERENCES

1. Brewer, Garry D. and Kakalik, James S., *Handicapped Children: Strategies for Improving Services*, McGraw-Hill, 1979.
2. Gliedman, John and Roth, William, *The Unexpected Minority: Handicapped Children in America*, Harcourt Brace Jovanovich, 1980.
3. Biklen, Douglas, *Let Our Children Go: An Organizing Manual for Advocates and Parents*, Human Policy Press, 1974.

4. Nelson, Roberta, *Creating Community Acceptance for Handicapped People*, Charles C. Thomas, 1978.
5. Pieper, Betty; Parent Papers: Advocacy, Art & Image.; Spina Bifida Assoc. of America (in process).
6. *How to Organize an Effective Parent Group and Move Bureaucracies*, Coordinating Council for Handicapped Children, Chicago, Illinois, 19 1971.

12
FINANCIAL CONCERNS

The question, "How can we pay for this?" may quickly follow on the heels of the initial parental reaction to a child's disability. A family that is just managing to cope with today's economic realities may be quite overwhelmed by the prospect of large, unplanned bills. The very integrity of the family's independence is threatened. Emotional reactions may subside, and families may be quite able to live with and enjoy the child; but the need for continuing treatment and specialized care may mean that financial anxieties may persist as far into the future as the family can see.

The issues involved in the costs of the provision of care and treatment need to be viewed from two perspectives. One of these is the individual family's struggle to cope with the financial demands of the disability. For families, this means both paying for the child's care and treatment now, in childhood, and of providing for the future security of both the child and the other members of the family. The pressures and the anxieties are both immediate and long-range. The family's ability to take care of itself financially forms an important part of its security and confidence. When this ability is threatened, the family may feel shaky indeed.

But the struggles exist not only within individual families. Some of the difficulties and uncertainties that families experience are the result of the inconsistent and ambiguous values of the larger society. Our society does not have a coherent answer to the question of who is responsible for the care, treatment, and education of children with special needs. Our approach is inconsistent at best; at worst, it is dishonest and unjust.

There is a child in Texas, now nine or ten years old, who has lived his entire life in a sterile, protected "bubble" because his body cannot fight disease. Each year as he has another birthday, news stories about him appear throughout the country. The stories seem to be positive, warm, and encouraging. Similarly, if an individual child's plight is brought to the attention of a community, this will often result in a massive outpouring of financial and emotional support for that child and the family. People tend to respond positively and generously to "real" people whose faces and stories they can learn about and identify with.

But when the question becomes whether we should provide such help and treatment for whole classes of children with birth defects or retardation, the answer is often different. Then, it seems, the cost is too great. It is easier to refuse anonymous groups of people than it is to deny a real, identifiable individual.

Our society has mixed feelings about the issue of who should bear the financial responsibility for the care and treatment of its members with special needs. Our values are in conflict. On the one hand, we tend to value independence of individuals and families, and to look favorably on those who can take care of themselves. On the other, we also have strong traditions of social programs to assist those in need. The wider social and philosophical questions of the meshing of individual responsibility, voluntary programs, and government assistance have not been clearly and rationally addressed.

The result is a hodgepodge of programs and services. Whether a particular family may be able to find financial assistance may depend on such factors as where they happen to live, where the parents work (what kind of insurance is provided by the employer), whether or not a voluntary organization exists for that specific condition, or whether that organization has funds or programs that the child needs.

The failure to address the underlying issues leads to gaps and inequities in programs that do exist. Whether a particular condition or disability qualifies a person or family for assistance depends on whether or not political pressure has been successfully applied in that area. Individual battles must be fought for each disability. Special Social Security provisions have been available for the blind, for example, but not for people with other disabilities. The Developmental Disabilities legislation has, in recent years, led to much tortuous discussion over which disabling conditions are to be included and which are not.

We seem to be unable to agree clearly on whether, and under what conditions, help is to be available. The many inconsistencies result in families being caught between programs, or not quite qualifying for those that do exist. Many families are angered and humiliated by being dependent on the whims of compassion and "charity."

Deeper values, and fears, may play a part in discussions held or the decisions that are made. These, however, are rarely mentioned overtly in legislative debates or hearings. These deeper values include questions about the value of human beings and human lives that are "different" in some way. The "quality of life" may be spoken about at times, but one is more likely to hear the discussion carried on in terms of cost-benefit analyses or other financial and economic terms. The fears are even deeper, and more infrequently voiced. These relate to the fear that our society may end up with too many people who are "defective," who will somehow drain or weaken the rest of us.

These are difficult questions and issues to face and resolve even if we could articulate them clearly and rationally. When they are hidden, however, they are all but impossible to address. We may hear the words, "There is not enough money for the program you need" and sense that underneath the message really is "We are afraid for ourselves of having too many people with your child's problem."

To the individual family seeking help for a child, these wider and deeper issues and questions may seem remote indeed. But they are not remote. They are part of the reason that the picture the parents find as they learn about services for their child is inconsistent, confusing, and sometimes unjust. Ours is a large and complex society, with many factors operating simultaneously. It is also not static. Trends and forces are constantly shifting and changing. Parents who cannot find what they need at first should not give up too quickly. Other approaches, other allies, or other methods with a better potential for success may exist now or in the near future.

The individual family with a child who needs expensive treatment faces an urgent and immediate problem. The costs of treatment with today's technology are high. Only the very wealthiest families can have any thought of absorbing these costs into their budgets. For the vast majority of families, help from somewhere will be essential. For some families who place a high value on self-sufficiency, asking for help for a child's care is difficult. It may seem like a failure. But it is simply not realistic to expect to be able to pay for unforeseen medical care which may cost thousands of dollars in a given year.

The two major sources of financial assistance are medical insurance and government aid. Private voluntary organizations and agencies form a third potential source of assistance. The picture, however, is inconsistent and uneven. Often it is the middle-income family, which can provide all normal expenses for itself but which cannot manage large medical bills, that finds the most difficulty. As Brewer and Kakalik write, "The rich have excellent medical services if they are willing to search them out and pay for them; and the poor, due mainly to the Medicaid and Crippled Children's programs, do have an institutional mechanism to which they can appeal for medical assistance for their handicapped children."[1] The people in middle, who can neither pay the costs themselves nor qualify for government aid, are often left stranded.

The financial assistance picture is uneven; it is also constantly changing as social pressures exert their influence. This means that families must not give up too easily. It is necessary to keep learning, asking, and looking, and, if they are not successful, to relearn, reask, and relook. Eventually, some families will face difficult choices. They may find that, in order to qualify for help or to find services, it is necessary to move, to change jobs, or to stay in a less desirable job because the insurance benefits are more complete. It is better, however, to face such choices squarely than not to know what they are.

HEALTH INSURANCE

Families with health insurance protection will need to become intimately familiar with the terms of their policies. Coverage terms will vary. There may be different limits for total benefits, benefits per year, or in the dollar amounts paid for hospital costs or physicians' fees. It is important that parents discuss the terms of their policies with people who are providing services. Sometimes, treatment can be timed to fit the policy's requirement, or negotiations can be arranged for the unpaid portion of the bills.

Some families will find that they are in effect trapped by a clause in a family health policy that excludes conditions diagnosed in the first week or 10 days of life. Policies containing this clause essentially exclude birth defects. Thus some families are misled into believing that they have a "family" health plan, only to discover that only family members who are born healthy and free of disabilities are covered. A number of states have made these clauses illegal.

Insurance benefits take on great importance when parents of children with disabilities consider changing jobs. The chance to pick up more coverage or major medical benefits (above and beyond basic protection) may well tip the scales in favor of a particular job. People who are thinking of changing coverage, however, need to check very carefully for any exclusions for "preexisting conditions." Families also need to be alert for any "open enrollment" opportunities, which are chances to enter into insurance programs without regard to physical examination or preexisting conditions.

Health insurance coverage for adults with disabilities who are no longer covered by their parents' policies may be a great problem. Some states, of which Wisconsin is one, are experimenting with risk-sharing plans for hard-to-insure people. In such a plan, all insurance carriers in the state are required to participate in order to share the risk. If only a few companies offered these policies, they would of course enroll all the people with disabilities who wanted coverage. This might pose a hardship which is not so likely if all companies are involved.

FEDERAL GOVERNMENT PROGRAMS

Government programs designed to provide assistance to individuals and families with special needs fall into two major categories: social insurance and public assistance. The basic philosophical approaches of insurance programs are different from those of programs of assistance. Government insurance programs, like private insurance, are based on a system of individuals paying into the program and receiving in return the eligibility to receive benefits when circumstances warrant them. Insurance programs thus are based on the person's having the designated condition or circumstances, and not on financial need. Examples of federal insurance programs include Medicare and Social Security Disability Insurance (SSDI).

Government assistance programs, on the other hand, are based on meeting financial eligibility requirements, and not on whether the person has paid into the system. Supplemental Security Income (SSI) is a prime example. This assistance is administered by the Social Security System, and provides a minimal monthly income for those whose disability prevents gainful employment. Children with disabilities may be eligible if their parents meet income requirements. For adults with disabilities, consideration for benefits is not dependent upon the income of the parents. Under certain conditions, disabled adults living with their parents may also qualify for SSI. Individuals and families can inquire about eligibility at their local Social Security office.

People with disabilities may also be entitled to Medical Assistance. SSI recipients are generally eligible for Medical Assistance as well as some housing subsidies. Benefits and services may vary considerably from state to state. This health care assistance program may pay for doctors' bills, hospital care, or for care in the home or in a private or public facility.

There is also a program called Medicaid Supplemental Care Assistance which some persons who are ineligible for SSI or Medical Assistance may qualify for. Some children with disabilities may also qualify if medical expenses exceed a given percentage of family income.

Other federal programs that may be of assistance to people with disabilities include rental subsidies under Section 8 of the Housing and Community Development Act and Title XX. The rental subsidies are available under Section 8 to individuals with disabilities who qualify by income and who are tenants of Housing and Urban Development Department approved housing. Title XX services include certain social and support services that contribute to self-care and self-support, and are also based on income eligibility rules.

At the time of this writing there is a great deal of uncertainty about the changes that may be made in government assistance programs and in eligibility requirements. Individuals and families will need to obtain current information from local or federal offices. One resource is a booklet entitled, "For the Disabled: A Pocket Guide to Federal Help," available from the Office for Handicapped Individuals, Room 338D, Humphrey Building, Washington, D.C. 20201.

STATE PROGRAMS

Assistance available through state-run programs is more variable. There may even be variations in eligibility requirements in different counties within the same state. Usually called Crippled Children's Services (CCS) (or some similar title), these programs provide assistance for medical treatment and the like. The funds available through these programs are limited to fixed amounts in a given year, so that these services cannot meet the total needs of the eligible population. According to Brewer and Kakalik, "CCS is reaching only a fraction of those who might benefit from it. Categorical coverage, as determined locally according to available resources and local preferences for certain classes of impairments over others, contributes to inequitable coverage from state to state and within the same state at different phases of the fiscal year."[1] These authors do feel, however, that this program does have some excellent features.

This variability means that families must do more seeking and more asking to learn what is available for them. In some states, (Wisconsin, for example), families must demonstrate to the director of county welfare or social services that "special circumstances," independent of income, do exist. Families are also well advised to contact other parents and parent organization to obtain information that others have already searched out and compiled. Individual families do not need to start from scratch in areas where other families and groups have already been involved.

VOLUNTARY ORGANIZATIONS

Voluntary organizations represent another category of potential assistance for some families which should not be overlooked. In addition to providing general information, referral, and emotional support there may be some direct financial assistance available, depending on the child's situation and the organization's policies. These policies and practices vary widely from organization to organization and sometimes within an organization depending upon the goals and programs of the local chapter.

Some voluntary organizations are concerned with the entire range of disabling conditions, whereas others concentrate on a specific disability. Even when parents find an organization for their child's disability, they should also contact the more broadly based ones to learn what might be available. These include organizations such as the National Foundation–March of Dimes and The National Easter Seal Society for Crippled Children and Adults (see Appendix A). Parents are also encouraged to write Closer Look, P.O. Box 1492, Washington, D.C. 20013, with questions about resources and services.

FEDERAL INCOME TAX

Parents of children with disabilities will want to familiarize themselves with regulations covering income tax deductions for expenses related to the child's care. This is being written at a time when substantial changes in the federal income tax are being considered, so that families will need to consult with their District IRS headquarters about specific questions that arise in the course of tax planning. Toll-free telephone numbers are available throughout the country for IRS district offices.

The Internal Revenue Service also has free literature available which may answer specific questions. Some useful booklets include the following.

Publication #17: Your Federal Income Tax
Publication #502: Deductions for Medical and Dental Expenses
Publication #503: Child Care and Disabled Dependent Care
Publication #526: Income Tax Deductions for Contributions

It is important to recognize that there are many individual variations in families' situations. Families may still have questions after reading these pamphlets. When this is the case, families can write to their local IRS office, explaining the situation and asking for a ruling on the matter.

Many families with children with disabilities spend substantial amounts on the child's care and treatment. Because these amounts often exceed the standard deductions allowed on the short tax form, it is often advantageous to file the longer form (1040) and itemize these deductions. While the specifics of dollar amounts for deductions may change, some general guidelines for planning for the preparation of federal income taxes will be likely to remain valid regardless of year-to-year changes. This section will focus on these guidelines. *The Exceptional Parent* magazine has in recent years published an annual "Tax Guide" for parents.[2] For information or reprints, parents may write to *The Exceptional Parent,* 296 Boylston Street, Boston, Massachusetts 02116.

Letting the IRS Know About the Situation

Income tax returns are processed by computers that automatically single out returns with unusual amounts for deductions. Therefore, a family filing a return with substantial amounts listed for deductions is more apt to be audited if the IRS has no knowledge of the individual situation. If, on the other hand, the IRS has an explanation of these high deductions, the personnel may understand the reasons for them and be less likely to pursue a complete audit.

How can a parent let the IRS know about the situation? This can be done by including a letter of explanation with the tax return. This letter should explain the disability and the reasons for the deductions claimed. A letter from the child's physician, documenting the disability and the treatments prescribed, is also useful. Parents should send copies of these letters with the completed tax forms and keep the originals in their files.

Keeping Records

Of critical importance in the matter of documenting expenditures is the keeping of records. This will be difficult for some families to organize, since expenses usually occur during periods of high stress for families. When the child is sick or is being transported for treatments, fittings, appointments, and the like, the family routine is disrupted and it may be difficult to remember to save and sort records and receipts. Parents who experience this difficulty may want simply to keep a large envelope or box labeled "Expenses" in a prominent place. If receipts are saved in this central place, they will be available for sorting and listing when time allows. A notebook, kept in this box or carried with the parent when keeping appointments, can help in recording items for which receipts are not given (such as travel expenses).

These records and receipts do not need to be submitted with the tax return, but they should be saved for three years after filing as IRS audits may be made for three years after that time. All bills, receipts, and cancelled checks relating to deductible expenses should be saved. If no formal receipt is given, the information about the item or service, the date, and the amount paid can be recorded on a piece of paper or in the notebook. Expenses are deductible for the year in which the payment is made. Thus if treatment was received in December of one

year, but the bill was paid in January of the next year, the expense is
deducted for the January date.

What is Deductible?

As *The Exceptional Parent* magazine explains, "The IRS definition
of medical care encompasses payments for the diagnosis, cure, allevia-
tion and treatment of disease or dysfunction of the body. In the
opinion of the IRS, anyone who renders services to diagnose, cure,
alleviate or treat a disease or dysfunction of the body qualifies as a
health care professional whose fees are deductible."[2] Thus the services
of many nonphysician professionals, such as occupational and physical
therapists, are deductible. In addition, special services rendered directly
to the disabled person such as by nurses, domestic help, or companions
may also be deductible. In some cases, payments for child care to relatives who are not also claimed as dependents may be deductible.

Special aids for the person with a disability are deductible when
they are obtained upon the advice of a doctor. These include a wide
range of items such as orthopedic appliances, lifting devices, special
telephone equipment, tape recorders, extra cost of a specially equipped
automobile, and remedial reading programs for dyslexic persons. Alter-
ations to a home that add to the value of the home are generally not
deductible. As *The Exceptional Parent* magazine explains, "For
example, if you install an elevator at a cost of $1,000 and the value
of your home is thus increased by $400, you may claim the difference,
$600, as a medical expense."[2]

Drugs and medications are also deductible expenses. Parents who
purchase over-the-counter medicines and supplies for their children may
deduct these, provided that they have been recommended by the child's
doctor for a specific reason. Special foods and beverages may also be
deducted when they are recommended by a physician and when their
cost is over and above that of a regular diet. If special foods are merely
substituted for what is normally consumed, the cost is not deductible.

Parents who have questions about whether or nor an item is deductible should contact the local IRS for information. The local office
can also advise as to the necessary documentation for these expenses.

Some education-related expenses are also deductible, such as the
cost of private schooling, if the primary purpose of that schooling is
for the treatment of that disability and if it has been recommended
by a practitioner. To qualify for deductions, such private schools
must offer specific programs for the treatment of the disability.
Recent IRS rulings have indicated that general benefits, such as a
healthy or beneficial atmosphere, are not enough to warrant deduc-
tion of costs of private schooling. Even when the child is receiving

a publicly funded educational program, additional expenses of the family related to education may be deductible. Examples of these might include costs of transporting the child to and from the school program or costs of additional classes that have been recommended.

Residential programs may also be deductible when they are part of a therapeutic program. For example, a home used to facilitate the transition from an institution to community living may qualify, whereas a home serving as a permanent residence may not (unless it is a licensed medical facility). Special camp costs are also deductible if recommended by the child's doctor, but not unless the camp has special facilities or programs relevant to the child's disability. As with school programs, camps are not deductible simply because attendance would be good for the child in general.

Travel expenses to and from medical care appointments and services are deductible. Families may wish to keep a separate notebook in the car to record dates, mileage, and expenses. If the child is being treated at a distant medical facility, the travel costs (but not the food and lodging) of one parent may be deductible if a doctor recommends the parent's presence as a medical necessity. Airfare or other travel expense for the child is always deductible.

Some educational or therapeutic expenses for parents that contribute to the child's treatment or health may be deductible. For example, if the doctor recommends that parents attend meetings of parent groups or educational programs, these may be deductible. However, the specific meeting must be educational or therapeutic and not simply social in order to qualify.

Again, parents are urged to remember that each family's individual situation is different. At any time of the year, families may write to the Ruling Department of the local IRS office, explaining the situation and the question and asking for a ruling on whether a particular expense is deductible or not. Accurate records, of course, are essential both in presenting the situation for ruling and in actually filing the tax returns.

LOOKING AHEAD

Future financial security, for the child with a disability and for the rest of the family, is a question that keeps many parents awake at night. The responsibility of providing adequately for the future of a child who might need extra assistance for a lifetime as well as for the parents' own retirement years may seem overwhelming. It takes courage to plan for the future; in order to plan, parents must allow themselves to face the possibilities and the uncertainties ahead. But it is through careful planning that parents may achieve the peace of mind which comes from knowing that they have done the best they could.

Each family's situation will be different, and there are no simple formulas for financial planning. Each family will need to weigh its own priorities; to see how these fit in with the assets available; and to determine how state laws and the availability of other sources of assistance affect the picture.

In terms of establishing priorities, most families will want to assure that assets are distributed fairly; that the needs of the nondisabled family members are taken into account as well as the special needs of the disabled member; and that the person with the disability has, if needed, a mechanism for assuring an advocate to protect his or her interests and rights. Some parents may feel that such planning is not useful because assets are limited. This is usually not true. Planning is still necessary in order to be sure that limited assets are used in the way that parents wish them to be. Some parents have found, for example, that assets which were to be held in trust for a child had to be used up before the child could qualify for state assistance.

Other parents may feel overwhelmed by the complexity of the financial situation and the need to collect so much information. Each parent does not need to start from scratch, however. Other people and groups have asked these questions, and parents can benefit from their experience. Local Associations for Retarded Citizens (ARC) are good resources for information about publications and names of attorneys who are well-versed in state laws as they relate to people with disabilities. Other advocacy and parent groups may also be helpful. Often, groups can invite people who are familiar with financial planning and state laws as guest speakers.

In addition to learning about how state and federal laws affect planning, the family will need to ask some questions about its own needs. These might include the following.

How expensive is the child's care?

How long will the care be needed?

How expensive is the equipment the child needs?

What is the child's potential in terms of education? What will the cost be?

How long will the child be dependent? (If the expectation is that the child will be likely to always be financially dependent, planning is very different than when the expectation is that he or she will be independent after age 22 or so.)

What benefits will the disabled person be eligible for?

What are the financial needs of the other children?

What are their educational needs?
Will the child with the disability be likely to need assistance in managing money or property?

For virtually all families, a will is essential. This is true even if the anticipated size of the estate is limited. If both parents die without leaving a will, the usual laws of the state apply. These laws do not ordinarily allow much flexibility for the consideration of specialized individual needs. Wills allow parents to make sure that their own wishes and intents are taken into account. Wills may also provide for the creation of trusts for all of the children, including the one with the disability. Parents will need to consult with an attorney who understands both the laws of the state and the wishes of the parents. Again, local groups such as ARC can help in providing names of such attorneys.

Life insurance is, for most families, a cornerstone of financial planning. Life insurance is both a protection against the loss of the parents' income before the children are grown, and the basis for the estate that the children can inherit. In most cases, the parents' primary concern is to provide funds for the child in the event that parents are no longer living or when the child is over 18. Thus it is most important that the parent have the life insurance, not the child. Generally, it is not recommended that the disabled son or daughter be named as beneficiary of parents' life insurance policies, because acquiring such an estate could make him or her ineligible for some financial assistance otherwise available. Parents should consult with their attorneys regarding trusts for the management of life insurance benefits. The major reasons to insure a child's life are to provide money for burial expenses or to guarantee future insurability. Future insurability is of course a factor when it is possible that the child will have dependents as an adult. For persons with some disabilities, insurability actually improves in later years because of medical advances. If parents should wish to insure the child's life, they may be able to participate in group plans offered by the National Association for Retarded Citizens (NARC) or other organizations.

Health insurance may be more of a problem for the person with a disability than life insurance when the youngster reaches the age of 19. NARC urges parents to be aggressive, and to continue to ask and apply.[3] There has been a great deal of activity in recent years in the area of health insurance for disabled adults. The National Association for Retarded Citizens is one group that has worked actively for state laws to provide that any permanently disabled child who is covered under a family or group plan continue to be eligible after the age of 19. Other states are experimenting with plans calling for all insurance carriers to participate in an insurance program for adults with disabilities.

People who have been denied coverage because of their disabilities
would be able to participate through this joint effort which reduces
the risk of the individual companies.

Parents of children who are retarded may wonder if their children
will be vulnerable to unscrupulous persons or need help in managing
money or property. Such parents may want to consider some form of
guardianship for the child. The question of guardianship is a complex
one; often the answer is not clear-cut. Since guardianships result in
total or partial loss of rights and decision-making powers, parents will
want to weigh carefully the best interest of the child. What is the
degree of risk for this child in terms of mismanagement of money or
harm to him or herself? Will the loss of rights be justified by the protection offered?

There are different types of guardianship possible. Total guardianship, called "plenary guardianship," involves complete supervision, with
loss of rights to vote, enter into contracts, give consent to surgery, or
marry without permission. This form, says the National Association for
Retarded Citizens, is unthinkable for a mildly retarded person.[3] Other
forms of limited or partial guardianship exist which do not involve a
judicial finding of incompetence. These may also allow the retarded
person to retain his or her rights, with the exception of any special
determinations that the person is incapable in specific areas.

The question of what person or persons should serve as the guard-
ian is also a difficult one. Potential or real conflicts of interest exist
in any form of guardianship, and these must be weighted carefully.
Brothers and sisters, for example, may sincerely have the well-being
of the retarded person at heart; but a conflict does exist if they have
a financial stake in the portion of the estate which would be left by
that retarded person's death. There are also disadvantages to having
banks or corporate trustees as sole managers. A financially conservative
attitude held by such trustees might lead them to reject expenditures
for the retarded person that the parents might have wished. Parents
who are considering guardianships can contact their local ARC for
assistance in finding suitable cotrustees. Some ARCs also have a common fund to help reduce the costs of trust management, especially
for small trusts where management costs seem out of proportion.

Although parents will want to plan carefully for their own assets
to be used in accordance with their wishes, the future financial security
for children with disabilities also depends on the network of resources
and programs available outside the family. Parents, parent groups, and
advocacy groups must continue to monitor existing programs and to
advocate to meet unmet needs. As NARC says,

"Real security for your son or daughter lies in appropriate quality education, vocational rehabilitation training, financial assistance through SSI, Medicaid, Social Security and other governmental benefits, appropriate quality residential living arrangements, state and federal legislation protecting the rights of retarded persons, advocacy programs which reach out to monitor and secure services to provide for retarded citizens the quality of life that all citizens deserve."[3]

QUESTIONS FOR PARENTS

1. Are the financial anxieties that I have about my child's care things that I can deal with?
2. Do I have enough information to be able to estimate what the costs will be?
3. Do I know where to look for guidance or assistance?
4. Do I have all the information I can get about: health insurance? government assistance? state programs? voluntary organizations?
5. Do I have a will which expresses my wishes and plans for the distribution of my estate?
6. Have I consulted with an attorney, as well as appropriate advocacy groups, about estate planning?
7. What about the needs of my nondisabled children? Are they taken into account?
8. Having planned as best I can, can I stop worrying unduly about the future?

REFERENCES

1. Brewer, Garry D. and Kakalik, James S., *Handicapped Children: Strategies for Improving Services*, McGraw-Hill, 1979.
2. 1980 Income Tax Guide, *The Exceptional Parent*, December 1980.
3. How to Provide for Their Future, National Association for Retarded Citizens, P.O. Box 6109, 2709 Avenue E. East, Arlington, Texas 76011.

13
WHEN HELP IS NEEDED

All families undergo change and stress with the passage of time. Children grow and must learn to cope with living in the world on their own; parents must learn to let them go and to prepare for their own aging. Factors in the outside world affect the family's sense of security and stability. Inflation, unemployment, and all of the social and economic problems that society faces touch the lives of families. As one set of problems or a developmental stage is managed and mastered, another appears to take its place.

The family's task is to cope with the demands of the outside world and at the same time to provide for a healthy and nurturing environment for the individuals within the family. According to Jerry M. Lewis, "a healthy family is one that does two things well: preserves the sanity and encourages the growth of parents and produces healthy children."[1] The psychological health of individual family members has a great deal to do with how the relationships within the family are functioning. People in families need to be free to be developing and autonomous individuals and also to be close and intimate with each other.

Psychological pain in families is expressed in a variety of ways. Children or teenagers may become excessively rebellious, or "act out"; parents may become depressed, overly anxious, or drink too much. A family member might become withdrawn and noncommunicative, or conflict and open fighting may become more frequent.

People in pain do not exist in isolation. The distress that is being expressed by the person with the "symptom" is also found, in one way or another, throughout the family. Relationships become tense and constricted; certain topics of conversation become forbidden, and freedom is curtailed. As Napier and Whitaker describe the troubled family, "[Family members] are so dependent on one another, so afraid of losing one another's support that in this fear they all agree intuitively not to 'rock the boat.' They fall into rigid patterns with one another, contriving intricate and tortuous routines that preserve their unity at the expense of their individuality."[2]

Things can, and do, happen in many families. Families do not need to have external stresses such as financial problems, poor health, accidents, or injuries to experience stress. This seems to be an obvious truth; and yet, it is often completely overlooked by families with a disabled member.

What happens all too frequently is that when the family of a child with a disability experiences stress or difficulty, it is assumed to be a natural part of the situation. For example, if a parent becomes depressed, he or she is likely to think, "Of course I feel depressed. How can I expect to feel otherwise, when I have the reality of my child's disability to cope with?" It usually does not occur to such a parent that he or she might be just as susceptible to the whole range of distress that humans can experience, quite apart from the disability of the child. And, since psychological help can obviously do nothing about the reality of the disability, the parent assumes that it can therefore do nothing to help relieve the distress.

That may not be the case at all. The easing of guilt or anger, or the development of different patterns of sharing the stresses, joys, and sorrows of the family's life may open up totally new ways of living with the same external reality. Individuals within the family may find that alternative ways of communicating with each other may help to make life less painful and more rewarding.

In previous generations the world was divided into two groups: the "sick" and the "well." The mentally ill were segregated into institutions often located far from their homes. Once a person was labelled as "sick" or "crazy," it was very difficult for him or her to overcome that label and to rejoin the "normal" world. Today, however, this is very different. A variety of forms of psychological help are available and it is much more socially acceptable to use them. One no longer has to be "crazy" to seek help; one only needs a desire to live better.

When a parent or family decides that perhaps psychological help would be useful in helping to find better ways of dealing with stress and problems, a new problem appears. A check of the Yellow Pages of most city telephone directories will show that many different types of therapy and therapists are available. Choosing a therapist who can be helpful can be a difficult matter.

TYPES OF THERAPY

Most people do not decide to seek professional help for emotional pain or adjustment problems until they are distressed enough to feel some urgency about their situation. It can be difficult for people to make thoughtful choices when they are upset and in crisis. Human responses and behaviors are a result of a complex meshing of internal reactions and external events. Psychological therapies approach the relief of emotional pain and distressing symptoms or behaviors in a variety of ways. Treatment may focus on the individual's understanding of the forces and motivations underlying his or her responses, on the behaviors causing distress, or on the relationships and communications of the people involved. Some basic knowledge about how these approaches differ may be helpful to the perplexed family.

Individual Psychotherapy

Individual psychotherapy has its roots in the traditional Freudian psychoanalytic approach. "Pure" psychoanalysis, in which a person is seen three to five times a week for the purpose of talking freely about his or her thoughts, dreams, and early memories, is rarely found today. Individual psychotherapy usually does, however, continue to focus on the person's search within himself for understanding or insights into why he acts and feels as he does. The assumption is that understanding the emotional roots of behaviors and conflicts will enable the person to change.

Indeed, this is often possible. The understanding and resolution of previously buried anger, fears, and guilt may allow a person freedom to experience new and more positive ways of living. Individual therapy is, however, often relatively lengthy. Sometimes, understanding one's responses and behaviors leads not to change but simply to a solidifying of "now I know *why* I am the way I am." However, sometimes changes in an individual cannot be maintained when the other people around that individual (members of the family system) continue to act in the old and powerful patterns.

Today, individual psychotherapy is likely not to be purely psychoanalytic, but rather, to be more psychosocial in nature. That is to say, the therapist takes into account not only knowledge about inner psychological development and mechanisms, but also the expanding body of knowledge about the relationships between individual experience and the nature and quality of interactions with other people and social forces. Individual therapy may encompass a wide variety of approaches. Therapists who prefer behavioral, Gestalt, or transactional analysis methods, for example, may work in one-to-one relationships with people.

Behavioral Therapies

Behavioral approaches assume that the essential emotional problem is visible and accessible through some aspect of the person's behavior.

The therapist begins by choosing an aspect of behavior to focus on, for example, fear or anxiety. The elements of that fearful response will be identified and clarified, as will the external situations that evoke the response. Behavioral therapy may include techniques of relaxation, desensitization, conditioning, and practice of new behaviors.

This focus of concentration on the specific behavior involved encourages a person to see "the problem" as something separate from his or her psychological self. The problem can thus be looked at, studied, and attacked without also attacking the basic sense of self that the person has. Behavioral therapy tends to be relatively brief and to engage the person very actively in trying out new approaches and responses.

Most behavioral therapies assume that when a behavior changes, so does a person's experience. When one acts differently, different things happen, both within oneself and in the responses of others. It is not necessary, according to these therapists, to understand the roots or the "whys" of the painful behaviors. Critics of the behavioral approach disagree. They maintain that if the distressing behavior is a result of underlying conflict that remains untouched, it is quite likely that another problem or symptom may take the place of the one that has been eliminated.

Social Therapies

A number of therapeutic approaches utilize the social dimensions of human experience, or how people react to and interact with each other. Many of these approaches involve people working with a therapist in groups instead of on an individual basis. Traditional group psychotherapy allows people not only to talk about how they relate to others but actually to experience those relationships in the therapy setting. Group therapy allows the observation and examination of actual responses to others without the added emotional "charge" of the original source of that pattern of response. For example, a person may relate to another group member in ways reminiscent of how he or she related to a father or mother.

Many other kinds of group therapy experiences may be available. The range of "group therapy" available may be quite perplexing. Groups may be offered for specific people or problems: returning veterans, abused wives, persons with sexual problems, gays, or people approaching retirement, to name just a few possibilities. Other groups are distinguished by their approaches. Gestalt therapy and transactional analysis are two approaches often used in group settings. In Gestalt therapy, conflicts within a person are not just talked about but are dramatized. People may act out, sometimes using different chairs, the different parts of themselves in conflict. A person might sit in one chair to speak as his conscience, for example, and another to speak as the part of himself that wants to rebel. Transactional analysis breaks down interactions between people into roles or "games." People react to each other as "child," "adult," or "parent," and the transaction between them can be analyzed in terms of which part they are speaking with and what "game" they are involved in.

Certainly there have been and will continue to be many innovations and fads in the group therapy field. As Joel Kovel says, "It would be hard to think of an approach to human life that has not found its way into the group setting and been called 'therapeutic', from multiple psychoanalysis to women's consciousness raising, satanism rituals, mass bioenergetic sessions, primals, nude marathons, and heaven knows what else."[3]

To complicate matters further for the person seeking help, therapists with any of these types of backgrounds can be found doing almost any type of therapy. Family therapists, for example, can be social workers, psychologists, or psychiatrists. While the training and credentials of a particular therapist will help to give some minimal assurance of competence, many other factors are necessary for a good therapeutic "match" of therapist and client. How then is the troubled person or family to know where to turn? Those seeking a group experience, particularly among the less traditional approaches, would be well-advised to learn as much as possible about the group and its leaders from both written materials and recommendations of others, both friends and professionals.

Family Therapy

The family approach to therapy has its roots in the assumption that human beings do not exist in isolation. People's feelings, behaviors, and experiences are not only a result of inner thoughts, motivations, and conflicts but are also intimately related to the nature of relationships and communications with others who are close. To a family therapist, it matters little what the symptom is or which member of the family is in trouble. The "problem" may appear as an acting-out child or as a wife's depression, but the family therapist will assume that this problem is related to pain and stress which is less obviously present in the way that the family lives and operates.

Family therapy's beginnings grew out of repeated observations that gains made in individual treatment often could not be maintained when the patient returned to the family setting. Or, if one member of a family succeeded in maintaining improvement, another family member, a spouse or another child, would begin to experience difficulty. Family therapy is a blending of understanding of an individual's inner world and the forces exerted upon individuals as they react together in the family system. When the entire family is present in the treatment room, the therapist does not need to spend a lot of time discussing with one person how the relationships and interactions work: he or she can hear and see the patterns as they happen. Thus family therapy may, depending on the nature of the problem and the goals of the family, be less lengthy than individual therapy.

Family therapy makes particular sense for members of families with a disabled member. Psychological pain is affected by the stresses of both internal conflicts and external relationships and events. While a child's disability may not "cause" a problem in another family member, it is certainly a fact of the family's life that must be dealt with and managed in some way. A distressed parent of a child with a disability may balk at family therapy, saying, "but I don't want my child to think that he or she is responsible for my problem."

However, a child who has had the opportunity openly to explore pain and stress as well as joy or love in therapy with the parents is probably less likely to feel responsible than a child who only observes a parent's unhappiness without this opportunity. Children tend to feel responsible for many events in family life. "If only I were a better child, Mommy and Daddy would not have gotten divorced" is a common response of childhood. Children who are present in therapy may be freed of these lonely and painful inferences, as well as receiving their own chance to acknowledge more openly their own feelings and reactions to being disabled.

Readers who would like to learn more about family therapy would do well to read *The Family Crucible* by Gus Napier with Carl Whitaker. An excellent review of the rationale for the family therapy is to be found in *A Complete Guide to Therapy: From Psychoanalysis to Behavior Modification* by Joel Kovel.

TRAINING OF THERAPISTS

To the person seeking help, it may seem as though there are almost as many types of therapists available as there are kinds of therapy. Psychiatrists, psychologists, and social workers can be found in abundance, as well as other counselors whose training and credentials may be less clear. The choice may be difficult; but it is also important. The decision to seek help is usually reached at a time when people feel upset, overwhelmed, and vulnerable. For growth to occur in therapy, there must be an atmosphere of mutual trust and respect between the therapist and the client or family, and it may not always be possible to know in advance that these will be present with a particular therapist.

Every competent therapist knows that his or her style and approach will not "fit" every person and every problem. If, after three or four sessions, the client or family feels that the necessary elements of trust and mutual respect are not present, it is perfectly appropriate to say "I don't feel that we are working well together." The competent therapist will not be hurt or threatened by this, and will often be able to help in making a more suitable referral. Too many people assume, if their first experience with therapy is not satisfactory, that therapy itself has failed. The truth is more likely to be that they had the misfortune to select a therapist who was not right for them.

Therapists have a variety of backgrounds and training. Good therapists come from all kinds of educational backgrounds; so do poor ones. While ultimately it will be the therapist's personality, commitment, and integrity that will probably be most critical, it may be useful to have some understanding of training backgrounds.

Psychiatrists

Psychiatrists are physicians, who have completed a medical school education before specializing in at least three additional years of psychiatric training. Thus psychiatrists have their grounding in general medicine, and are well-equipped to differentiate between physical and emotional components of distress. As physicians, they are able to utilize a wide range of therapeutic measures, including the prescribing of medication and hospitalization, when this is advisable. There may be fewer problems with insurance coverage if the therapist has an M.D. or when there is medical supervision of the nonmedical therapist. Although medical school training does encourage physicians to think in terms of "sickness" and "health," many psychiatrists are also well-grounded in social and family systems approaches to human distress.

Psychologists

Most therapists with doctoral degrees in psychology are well-grounded in personality development. While some have backgrounds in experimental psychology, most have also had clinical experience and at least as much, if not more, training in psychological and social factors than psychiatrists.

Social Workers

The training of social workers may be more varied than that of psychiatrists or psychologists. Some will have had a great deal of work in social policy and social agencies. Most social workers who are therapists have had training and supervised experience in psychological treatment. Therapists who are social workers may have either a master's degree (M.S.W.) or a doctorate (Ph.D.). A social work background is especially helpful in understanding how a variety of family and social forces influence an individual's experience.

Others

Therapists may also be psychiatric nurses with advanced training and may work in social or mental health agencies or in private practice. Other therapists may come from a variety of original backgrounds, but for the most part families should look for a therapist with a degree in one of the mental health or psychological fields.

CHOOSING A THERAPIST

There are, unfortunately, no guarantees that the first therapist a person chooses will be "right" or helpful. The client's own instincts and judgments about the therapist's concern and respect for the client's integrity will be at least as important as any licences or credentials the therapist may have. Since these elements cannot be evaluated until people have actually met a therapist, other sources of information will be needed to make a selection.

Recommendations from others who are more knowledgeable are important guides to a therapist's reputation. Trusted friends, physicians, or other professional people who have been involved in caring for the child with a disability may be helpful in learning about therapists and resources in the community. Whether a family seeks help through someone in private practice or through a mental health agency will depend on the availability of insurance or other assistance in paying for these services.

Some mental health or family service agencies can provide excellent psychological services, often on a sliding-scale basis in which fees are adjusted according to the family's income. Medical Assistance does cover some mental health treatment, although this is more variable and may change depending on budgetary and political pressures in the state. People entering treatment should investigate their insurance coverage or other assistance carefully and not hesitate to speak frankly with the prospective therapist about the subject of payment for treatment.

For many specific kinds of problems, low-cost programs and support groups may be available in the community. Alcohol and drug abuse programs, services for abused women and children, or teen-age rap centers are but a few examples. Most of these will provide information about their programs to anonymous telephone callers.

The family of a child with a disability may feel that it is necessary to find a therapist who is knowledgeable about that specific disability. In most cases, this is not so. The family can tell the therapist what he or she needs to know about the disability and its effects. It is far more important that the therapist be knowledgeable about family systems, how they operate, and the effects of stress upon individuals and families. The therapist is not going to treat the disability itself: that is the job of the other professionals involved with the child. The therapist's task is to help the family to cope with its stresses and to provide a creative and nurturing environment for each of the family members.

Each family must decide for itself whether the quality of its life together is satisfactory or whether it may be possible to find a greater level of comfort of family members. The problem is that most of us only "know" what we have already experienced in our current families and the families we grew up in.

Obvious "symptoms" — such as severe depression in a parent, or disturbed behavior in a child — may serve as a catalyst for change in much the same way that stomach pain motivates a person to get treatment for ulcers. Quiet pain, or living a life at a less than optimal level, may be more difficult for a family to recognize. Family members may simply assume that this is "the way life is." Or, people may turn to alcohol, drugs, excessive preoccupation with work, or extramarital affairs to search for additional zest or peace in their lives. Our families are truly where we live and flourish; the quality of that life deserves our most careful attention.

QUESTIONS FOR PARENTS

Questions about how the family is living and how the family members are faring both in relationships with each other and outside the home need to be asked from time to time. Such a "family check-up" might include the following areas.

1. How well is the family managing the tasks of living and the pursuit of its goals?
2. Can family members share their thoughts and feelings with each other?
3. Can each member find satisfaction in school, work, or friendships outside the home?

4. Can the parents enjoy each other as partners and lovers as well as coparents?
5. Can family members both fight and play with each other?
6. Does each person have a sense of his or her own individual identity as well as an identity as a member of the family?

REFERENCES

1. Lewis, Jerry M., *How's Your Family? A Guide to Identifying Your Family's Strengths and Weaknesses*, Brunner-Mazel, 1979.
2. Napier, Gus, and Whitaker, Carl, *The Family Crucible*, Harper and Row, 1978.
3. Kovel, Joel, *A Complete Guide to Therapy: From Psychoanalysis to Behavior Modification*, Pantheon Books, 1976.

Appendix A
ORGANIZATIONS

The following are some sources of information on handicapping conditions and organizations. Parents or others who are experiencing difficulty in locating an appropriate organization because it is not listed in this appendix or because the address is out of date may wish to consult some of these sources.

Closer Look, Box 1492, Washington, D.C. 20013.

Council for Exceptional Children, 1920 Association Drive, Reston, Virginia 22091.

The Directory of Organizations Interested in the Handicapped, People-to-People Committee for the Handicapped, 1522 K Street N.W., Suite 1130, Washington, D.C. 20005. $2.00 for persons with disabilities and families, $3.00 to others.

The Exceptional Parent, 296 Boylston Street, Third Floor, Boston, Massachusetts 02116,

National Easter Seal Society, 2023 West Ogden Avenue, Chicago, Illinois 60612, or contact local branch.

National Foundation–March of Dimes, 1275 Mamaroneck Avenue, White Plains, New York 10605.

Resource Directory; Directory of National Information Sources on Handicapping Conditions and Related Services, published by the Office for Handicapped Individuals, Office of Human Development Services, Department of Education. Publication number DHEW (OHDS) 80-22007, cost, $6.50. Write: Superintendent of Documents, U. S. Government Printing Office, Washington, D. C. 20402.

ALPHABETICAL LISTING OF ORGANIZATIONS

Alexander Bell Association for the Deaf
3417 Volta Pl., N.W.
Washington, D.C. 20007

American Association for the Education of the Severely/Profoundly
Handicapped
1600 West Armory Way
Seattle, Washington 98119

American Association on Mental Deficiency
5201 Connecticut Ave., N.W.
Washington, D.C. 20015

American Foundation for the Blind
15 West 16th Street
New York, New York 10011

American Speech and Hearing Association
10801 Rockville Pike
Rockville, Maryland 20852

Amyotrophic Lateral Sclerosis Society of America
15300 Ventura Blvd. Suite 315
P.O. Box 5951
Sherman Oaks, California 91403

Arthritis Foundation
3400 Peachtree Rd. N.E. Suite 1101
Atlanta, Georgia 30326

Arthrogryposis Association, Inc.
106 Herkimer Street
North Bellmore, New York 11710

Association for Children with Learning Disabilities
4156 Library Avenue
Pittsburgh, Pennsylvania 15234

Association for the Education of the Visually Handicapped
919 Walnut Street, Fourth Floor
Philadelphia, Pennsylvania 19107

Association for Retarded Citizens
National Headquarters
2709 Avenue E, East
Arlington, Texas 76011

Association for the Visually Handicapped
1839 Frankfort Avenue
Louisville, Kentucky 40206

Council for Exceptional Children
1920 Association Drive, Dept. 3108
Reston, Virginia 22091

Cystic Fibrosis Foundation
6000 Executive Blvd., Suite 309
Rockville, Maryland 20852

Down's Syndrome Congress
706 S. Bunn Street
Bloomington, Illinois 61701

The Dysautonomia Foundation
370 Lexington Avenue, Room 1508
New York, New York 10017

Epilepsy Foundation of America
1828 L Street N.W.
Washington, D.C. 20036

Friedrich's Ataxia Group in America
P.O. Box 11116
Oakland, California 94611

International Association of Parents of the Deaf
814 Thayer Avenue
Silver Spring, Maryland 20910

Juvenile Diabetes Foundation
23 E. 26th Street
New York, New York 10010

League for Emotionally Disturbed Children
171 Madison Avenue
New York, New York 10017

Little People of America
P.O. Box 126
Owatonna, Minnesota 55060

Muscular Dystrophy Association, Inc.
810 Seventh Avenue
New York, New York 10019

National Aid to the Visually Handicapped
3201 Balboa Street
San Francisco, California 94121

National Association for the Deaf
814 Thayer Avenue
Silver Spring, Maryland 20970

National Association for Down's Syndrome
170 N. Harvey
Oak Park, Illinois 60302

National Association for the Visually Handicapped
305 E. 24th Street, 17-C
New York, New York 10010

National Easter Seal Society for Crippled Children and Adults
2023 W. Ogden Avenue
Chicago, Illinois 60612

National Foundation–March of Dimes
1275 Mamaroneck Avenue
White Plains, New York 10605

National Hemophelia Foundation
25 West 39th Street
New York, New York 10018

National Multiple Sclerosis Society
205 E. 42nd Street
New York, New York 10017

National Society for Autistic Children
1234 Massachusetts Avenue, N.W. Suite 1017
Washington, D.C. 20005

National Tay-Sachs and Allied Diseases Association
122 E. 42nd Street
New York, New York 10017

Osteogenesis Imperfecta, Inc.
632 Center Street
Van Wert, Ohio 45891

Spina Bifida Association of America
343 South Dearborn, Suite 317
Chicago, Illinois 60604

United Cerebral Palsy Associations
66 East 34th Street
New York, New York 10016

United Ostomy Association
2001 W. Beverly Blvd.
Los Angeles, California 90057

ORGANIZATIONS CONCERNED WITH LEGAL RIGHTS

ABA Mental Disability Legal Resource Center
1800 M Street N.W.
Washington, D.C. 20036

American Civil Liberties Union (ACLU)
85 Fifth Avenue
New York, New York 10011

American Coalition for Citizens with Disabilities
1200 15th Street N.W. Suite 201
Washington, D.C. 20005

Architectural and Transportation Barriers Compliance Board
Mary Switzer Memorial Bldg. Suite 1010
Washington, D.C. 20201

Center for Law and the Deaf
Seventh and Florida Avenues, Northeast
Washington, D.C. 20002

Children's Defense Fund
1520 New Hampshire Avenue, N.W.
Washington, D.C. 20036

Committee for the Handicapped People-to-People Program
La Salle Building, Suite 610
Connecticut Avenue and L Street
Washington, D.C. 20036

Coordinating Council for Handicapped Children
407 S. Dearborn
Chicago, Illinois 60605

National Center for Child Advocacy
P.O. Box 1182
Washington, D.C. 20013

National Committee for Children and Youth
1145 19th Street, Northwest
Washington, D.C. 20009

President's Committee on Employment of the Handicapped
1111 20th Street N.W. 6th Floor
Washington, D.C. 20210

President's Committee on Mental Retardation
Seventh and D Streets, S.W.
Washington, D.C. 20201

Untapped Resources, Inc. (Legal Services)
60 First Avenue
New York, New York 10009

ORGANIZATIONS FOR RECREATION

American Blind Bowling Association, Inc.
150 N. Bellaire Avenue
Louisville, Kentucky 40206

American Wheelchair Bowling Association, Inc.
2424 N. Federal Highway Suite 109
Boynton Beach, Florida 33435

Blind Outdoor Leisure Development
533 E. Main
Aspen, Colorado 81611

The National Association of Sports for Cerebral Palsy
P.O. Box 3874
Amity Station, New Haven, Connecticut 06525

National Council for Therapy and Rehabilitation Through Horticulture
Mount Vernon, Virginia 22121

National Therapeutic Recreation Society
Branch of National Recreation and Park Association
1601 N. Kent Street
Arlington, Virginia 22209

National Wheelchair Basketball Association
Office of the Commissioner
110 Seaton Bldg.
University of Kentucky
Lexington, Kentucky 40506

North American Riding for the Handicapped Association
Box 100
Ashburn, Virginia 22011

United States Deaf Skiers Association
159 Davis Avenue
Hackensack, New Jersey 07601

The Wheel Chair Motorcycle Association, Inc.
101 Torrey Street
Brockton, Massachusetts 02401

Winter Park Handicapped Ski Program
Box 313
Winter Park, Colorado 80482

Appendix B
BIBLIOGRAPHY

There has been a dramatic increase in recent years in publications written about disabilities in children. It is not possible in this listing to include all such books and pamphlets, nor to hope to address all the specific needs that readers may have. The suggestions that follow are but a sampling of resources that exist; for the most part, they are addressed primarily to parents and this author has found them useful.

Parents who wish to read more need not necessarily spend large sums of money on books. Many of these are available in public libraries, or may be owned by local branches of organizations and parent groups willing to loan them out. Borrowing books for review can enable parents to decide which of them are relevant to their own individual situations. Many of the books listed contain their own listings of further resources.

There are several sources of more comprehensive listings of books and resources, including a wealth of titles on specific disabilities and their management. Readers may wish to contact the following to obtain further information on written materials available:

The Exceptional Parent Bookstore, 296 Boylston Street 3rd Floor, Boston, Massachusetts 02116. Offers a variety of general and specific books and articles. Ask for a listing of titles and ordering information.

A Reader's Guide: For Parents of Children with Mental, Physical, or Emotional Disabilities. By Coralie B. Moore and Kathryn Gorham Morton, with the assistance of Joni B. Mills. Publication #(HSA) 77-5290, from Public Health Service, Health Services Administration, Bureau of Community Health Services, Rockville, Maryland

20857. This is a comprehensive list of books, resources, and organizations complete with addresses and prices.

RESOURCES

General

Ayrault, Evelyn West. *You Can Raise Your Handicapped Child.* New York: G.P. Putnam's Sons, 1964.

Ayrault, Evelyn West. *Helping the Handicapped Teenager Mature.* New York: Association Press, 1971.

Brown, Sara L. and Moersch, Martha (Eds.). *Parents on the Team.* Ann Arbor: University of Michigan Press, 1978.

Doyle, Phyllis B., Goodman, John F., Grotsky, Jeffrey N. and Mann, Lester. *Helping the Severely Handicapped Child: A Guide for Parents and Teachers.* Thomas Y. Crowell, 1979.

Featherstone, Helen. *A Difference in the Family: Life with a Disabled Child.* New York: Basic Books, Inc., 1980.

Gordon, Sol. *Living Fully: A Guide for Young People with a Handicap, Their Parents, Their Teachers, and Professionals.* New York: John Day Co., 1975.

Heisler, Verda. *A Handicapped Child in the Family: A Guide for Parents.* New York: Grune & Stratton, 1972.

McDonald, Eugene T. *Understand Those Feelings: A Guide for Parents of Handicapped Children and Everyone Who Counsels Them.* Pittsburgh: Stanwix House, 1962.

McCleary, Elliott H. and Denhoff, Eric. Your Child Has a Future (Booklet). Chicago: National Easter Seal Society for Crippled Children and Adults, 1978.

McNamara, Joan and McNamara, Bernard. *The Special Child Handbook.* New York: Hawthorne Books, 1977.

Pieper, Elizabeth. *When Something is Wrong with Your Baby: Looking In and Reaching Out.* (Booklet). Spina Bifida Association of America, 343 S. Dearborn, Chicago, Illinois 60604. 1977. ($1.00)

Stigen, Gail K. *Heartache and Handicaps: An Irreverent Survival Manual for Parents.* Palo Alto: Science and Behavior Books, 1976.

Wentworth, Elise H. *Listen to Your Heart: A Message to Parents of Handicapped Children.* Houghton Mifflin, 1974.

Zuckerman, Lawrence, and Yura, Michael T. *Raising the Exceptional Child: Meeting the Everyday Challenges of the Handicapped or Retarded Child.* New York: Hawthorne Books, 1979.

Periodicals

The Exceptional Parent
296 Boylston Street, Third Floor
Boston, Massachusetts 02116 ($14 per year to individuals)

Accent on Living
P.O. Box 700
Gillum Road and Hugh Drive
Bloomington, Illinois 61701 ($4.00 per year)

More Specific

Blodgett, Harriet. *Mentally Retarded Children: What Parents and Others Should Know.* Boston: University of Minnesota Press, 1971.

Brutten, Milton; Richardson, Sylvia and Mangel, Charles. *Something's Wrong with My Child: A Parent's Book about Children with Learning Disabilities.* New York: Harcourt, Brace and World, 1973.

Cunningham, Cliff and Soper, Patricia. *Helping Your Exceptional Baby: A Practical and Honest Approach to Raising a Mentally Handicapped Child.* New York: Pantheon Books.

Finnie, Nancie. *Handling the Young Cerebral Palsied Child at Home.* New York: E.P. Dutton, 1975.

Gardner, Richard A., M.D. *The Family Book About Minimal Brain Dysfunction.* New York: Jason Aronson, 1973.

Logue, Patrick E. *Understanding and Living with Brain Damage.* Springfield, Illinois: Charles C. Thomas, 1975.

Myklebust, Helmer. *Your Deaf Child: A Guide for Parents.* Springfield, Illinois: Charles C. Thomas, 1979.

Riesz, Elizabeth Durkman. *First Years of a Down's Syndrome Child,* Special Child Publications, 4535 Unioh Bay Place, N.E., Seattle, Washington 98105.

Rosner, Jerome. *Helping Children Overcome Learning Difficulties: A Step-By-Step Guide for Parents and Teachers.* New York: Walker & Co., 1975.

Siegel, Ernest. *The Exceptional Child Grows Up: Guidelines for Understanding and Helping the Brain-Injured Adolescent and Young Adult.* New York: E.P. Dutton, 1974.

Swinyard, Chester. *The Child with Spina Bifida.* (Booklet). Spina Bifida Association of America, 343 S. Dearborn, Chicago 60604. Revised 1979. ($1.00)

White, Robin. *The Special Child: A Parent's Guide to Mental Disability*. Boston: Little, Brown, 1978.

For Children

Altshuler, Anne. Books That Help Children with a Hospital Experience. U.S. Government Printing Office, Washington, D.C. 20402. Publication (HSA) 74-5402. 1974.

Fassler, Joan. *One Little Girl*. New York: Human Sciences Press, 1969 How a "slow" child can be fast at some things (ages 3 to 8).

Grealish, MaryJane Van Braunsberg and Grealish, Charles A. *Amy Maura*. Syracuse: Human Policy Press, 1975. About a girl with cerebral palsy and the day she is a heroine. Also about the self-concept of a child with a handicap (primarily for ages 8 and younger).

Larsen, Hanne. *Don't Forget Tom*. New York: Crowell, 1978. A 6-year-old has trouble keeping up because part of his brain doesn't work; his brother and sister encourage and help him.

Little, Jean. *Mine for Keeps*. Boston: Little, Brown, 1962. A child with cerebral palsy adjusts to life at home after a special school (ages 9 to 12).

Savitz, Harriet May. *Fly, Wheels, Fly*. New York: John Day, 1970. Two teenagers in wheelchairs learn about themselves through sports (ages 9 to 14).

Stein, Sara Bonnett. *About Handicaps*. New York: Walker & Co., 1974. Friendship between two boys, one with cerebral palsy (for young children).

Wolf, Bernard. *Don't Feel Sorry for Paul*. Philadelphia: Lippincott, 1974. An active 7-year-old boy with leg and arm prostheses.

Wrightson, Patricia. *A Race Course for Andy*. New York: Harcourt, Brace Jovanovich, 1968. A boy's efforts to keep up with his friends (ages 9 to 14).

For Siblings

Baldwin, Anne. *A Little Time*. New York: Viking, 1978. The 10-year-old narrator, Sarah, tells of the difficulties and rewards of a younger retarded brother.

Byars, Betsy. *Summer of the Swans*. New York: Viking, 1970. The ambivalent feelings of an adolescent girl for her younger retarded brother.

Clearly, Margaret. *Please Know Me as I Am: A Guide to Helping Children Understand the Child with Special Needs.* Sudbury, Pennsylvania: Jerry Clearly, 1975.

Heide, Florence Parry. *Sound of Sunshine, Sound of Rain.* Bergenfield, New Jersey: Parent's Magazine Press, 1970. The special world of the blind child (ages 5 to 8).

Lasker, Joe. *He's My Brother.* Chicago: Whitman, 1974. A brother's love and impatience with his handicapped sibling.

Levine, Edna S. *Lisa and Her Soundless World.* New York: Human Sciences Press, 1974. To help a hearing child comprehend a world without sound (ages 5 to 8).

Luis, Earlene and Millar, Barbara F. *Listen, Lissa.* New York: Dodd, Mead & Co., 1968. The joys and problems of the family of a severely retarded boy.

Peterson, Jeanne Whitehouse. *I Have a Sister: My Sister is Deaf.* New York: Harper & Row, 1979 (for younger children).

Sobol, Harriet. *My Brother Steven is Retarded.* New York: Macmillan & Co., 1977. A 7-year-old girl's feelings about and experiences with her older retarded brother.

For Teens

Ayrault, Evelyn West. *Helping the Handicapped Teenager Mature.* New York: Association Press, 1964.

Gordon, Sol. *Living Fully: A Guide for Young People with a Handicap, Their Parents, Their Teachers, and Professionals.* New York: John Day Co., 1975.

Mitchell, Joyce Slayton. *See Me More Clearly: Career Planning for Teens with Physical Disabilities.* New York: Harcourt, Brace Janovich, 1980.

Pieper, Elizabeth. *By, For and With ... Young Adults with Spina Bifida. Spina Bifida Association of America, 343 S. Dearborn, Chicago, Illinois 60604, 1979 ($1.00).*

ADVOCACY

Biklen, Douglas. *Let Our Children Go: An Organizing Manual for Advocates and Parents.* Syracuse, New York: Human Policy Press, 1974.

Brewer, Garry D. and Kakalik, James S. *Handicapped Children: Strategies for Improving Services.* New York: McGraw-Hill, 1979.

Consent Handbook. American Association on Mental Deficiency, 5101 Wisconsin Avenue, N.W., Washington, D.C. 20016.

Gliedman, John and Roth, William. *The Unexpected Minority: Handicapped Children in America.* For the Carnegie Council on Children. New York: Harcourt, Brace, Jovanovich, 1980.

Hall, Kent. *The Rights of Physically Handicapped People.* New York: Avon, Books.

How to Organize an Effective Parent Group and Move Bureaucracies. Coordinating Council for Handicapped Children, 407 S. Dearborn, Chicago, Illinois 60605, 1971.

Nelson, Roberta. *Creating Community Acceptance for Handicapped People.* Springfield, Illinois: Charles C. Thomas, 1978.

Producing a Public Relations Program for Disabled Adults. President's Committee on Employment of the Handicapped, Washington, D.C. 20210.

Wolfensberger, Wolf. *The Principle of Normalization in Human Services.* National Institute on Mental Retardation, Kinsmen NIMR Bldg., York University Campus, 4700 Keele Street, Downsview, Toronto, Ontario M3J 1P3, 1972.

EDUCATION

Adams, Howard. Parent's Guide to the Education for All Handicapped Children Act. Spina Bifida Association of Greater Kansas City, P.O. Box 5462, Kansas City, Missouri 64131.

Due Process and the Exceptional Child in Pennsylvania: A Guide for Parents, Education Law Center, Inc., 2100 Lewis Tower Bldg., 225 South 15th Street, Philadelphia, Pennsylvania 19102. Single copies free. (Written for Pennsylvania. This has much information useful to parents in other states as well.)

How to Prepare for a Due Process Hearing. Coordinating Council for Handicapped Children, 407 S. Dearborn Rm. 680, Chicago, Illinois 60605 (reprint).

Klein, Stanley. *Psychological Testing of Children: A Consumer's Guide.* Boston: The Exceptional Parent Press, 1977.

Mainstreaming: A Comprehensive View. Exceptional Parent Bookstore, 296 Boylston Street, Boston, Massachusetts 02116 (reprints).

Pieper, Betty. The Teacher and the Child with Spina Bifida. Spina Bifida Association of America, 343 S. Dearborn, Chicago, Illinois 60604. Revised 1979 ($1.00)

SBAA Fact Information Booklet: Special Education. Spina Bifida Association of America, 343 S. Dearborn, Chicago, Illinois 60604.

Sontag, E. (Ed.). *Educational Programming for the Severely and Profoundly Handicapped.* Council for Exceptional Children, 1920 Association Drive, Reston, Virginia 22091.

EQUIPMENT

General

Accent on Living: Buyer's Guide. Information on products for the disabled. Updated every two years. Cheever Publishing, Inc., P.O. Box 700, Bloomington, Illinois 61701.

Bruck, Lilly. *Access: The Guide to a Better Life for Disabled Americans.* Becoming a more knowledgeable consumer and locating special products. Random House Mail Service, 201 E. 50th Street, New York, New York 10022.

Hale, Glorya (Ed.) *Source Book for the Disabled.* Paddington Press.

Hofmann, Ruth B. *How to Build Special Furniture for Handicapped Children.* Springfield, Illinois: Charles C. Thomas, 1974.

Robinault, Isabel P. *Functional Aids for the Multiply Handicapped.* New York: Harper & Row, 1973.

Clothing

Clothing Designs for the Handicapped. Accent Special Publications, Box 700, Bloomington, Illinois 61701. Designs, instructions, and directions for altering clothing and patterns ($15.00).

Clothing for Handicapped People. President's Committee on Employment of the Handicapped, 1111 20th Street N.W., Washington, D.C. 20210. Includes information on services and manufacturers who sell shoes in different sizes.

Fashion-Able. Rocky Hill, New Jersey 08553. Catalogues of self-help items, books and clothing.

Self-Help Clothing for Children Who Have Physical Disabilities. By Eleanor Boettke Hotte. National Easter Seal Society, 2023 West Ogden Avenue, Chicago, Illinois 60612 ($1.50 plus 75¢ postage and handling).

Catalogues

It is beyond the scope of this book for this author to have personally investigated the manufacturers and products listed here. These listings are suggested as starting points for the collecting of information; parents will need to weigh carefully the special needs of the child, the cost of the items, professional advice, and their own common sense in making purchases. These companies provide catalogues upon request.

AAMED, Inc.
1215 S. Harlem Avenue
Forest Park, Illinois 60130

Abbey Rents and Sells
13500 S. Figueroa
Los Angeles, California 90061

Adaptive Therapeutic Systems, Inc.
162 Ridge Road
Madison, Connecticut 06443

Amigo
6693 S. Dixie Highway
Bridgeport, Michigan 48722 (3-wheeled motorized wheelchairs)

Cleveland Orthopedic Company
3957 Mayfield Avenue
Cleveland, Ohio 44121

Equipment Shop
P.O. Box 33
Bedford, Massachusetts 01730
(Send large self-addressed, stamped envelope)

Genac, Inc.
2220 Norwood Avenue
Boulder, Colorado 80302 (Pogon buggy)

The Independence Factory
Fred Carroll
1385 Central Avenue
Middletown, Ohio 45042
(Develops and manufactures self-help devices, many made from low-cost factory-reject materials. Will try to assist with design problems.)

Invacare
1200 Taylor Street
Elyria, Ohio 44035

Lossing Company
2217 Nicollet Avenue
Minneapolis, Minnesota 55404
(Manufactures the Row car for young children)

Maddak, Inc.
Industrial Road
Pequannock, New Jersey 07440

Medical Equipment Distributors, Inc.
1701 S. First Avenue
Maywood, Illinois 60153

Modular Medical Corp.
177 E. 88th Street
New York, New York 10028

Mulholland and Associates
1563 Los Angeles Avenue
Ventura, California 93003 (growth guidance chairs)

Ortho-Kinetics
P.O. Box 2000 JOT 106
Waukesha, Wisconsin 53186 (care chairs)

Prentke Romick Company
Box 191 P
Shreve, Ohio 44676 (electronic communication aids)

Rehabilitation Equipment, Inc.
1556 Third Avenue
New York, New York 10028

Rifton Equipment for the Handicapped
Rifton, New York 12471

Telesensory Systems, Inc.
3408 Hillview Avenue
P.O. Box 10099
Palo Alto, California 94304 (communication aids)

Voyager, Inc.
P.O. Box 1577
South Bend, Indiana 46634 (battery-operated chair)

FINANCIAL

Dickinson, Peter A. and the editors of *Consumer Guide. Getting Your Share.* Publications International, Ltd., 3841 W. Oakton Street, Skokie, Illinois 60076.

For the Disabled — A Pocket Guide to Federal Help. Office for Handicapped Individuals, Room 338D, Humphrey Building, Washington, D.C. 20201.

Garrett, Jon R. Planning A More Secure Future. Michigan Association for Retarded Citizens, 416 Michigan National Tower, Lansing, Michigan 48933.

How to Provide for Their Future. National Association for Retarded Citizens, P.O. Box 6109, 2709 Avenue E, East, Arlington, Texas 76011.

Income Tax Guide. The Exceptional Parent, 296 Boylston Street, Boston, Massachusetts 02116.

Information on Tax Deductions. Coordinating Council for Handicapped Children, 407 S. Dearborn, Chicago, Illinois 60605 (free with stamped, self-addressed envelope).

The Name of the Game is Economics. Reprints from the Exceptional Parent. # S-131. Exceptional Parent Bookstore, 296 Boylston Street, Boston, Massachusetts 02116 ($2.50).

Social Security Handbook. Available from local office or Superintendent of Documents, Washington, D.C. 20201 (Pub. # DHEW SSA-73-10135) ($4.30 plus $1 for mailing).

SSI Advocates Handbook. Center on Social Welfare Policy and the Law, 95 Madison Avenue, New York, New York 10016.

Supplemental Security Income for Retarded People. Superintendent of Documents, Washington, D.C. 20201 (Pub. # SSA 76-11050).

GENETICS

Books

Henden, David and Marks, Joan. *The Genetic Connection.* New York: William Morrow & Co., 1978.

Milunsky, Aubrey M. *Know Your Genes.* New York: Houghton Mifflin, 1977.

BROCHURES

Genetic Counseling. National Foundation–March of Dimes, Box 2000, White Plains, New York 10602.

Can Genetic Counseling Help You? National Genetics Foundation, 9 West 57th Street, New York, New York 10019.

HOUSING AND RESIDENTIAL ISSUES

A Place of Our Own: Tips for Mentally Retarded People Living in the Community. (11 pp.) The President's Committee on Employment of the Handicapped, Washington, D.C. 20210.

Cole, Jean A., Sperry, Jane C. and Board, Mary Ann. *New Options.* TIRR, 1333 Moursund Avenue, Houston, Texas 77030 ($3.95).

Developing Alternative Residential Services for the Multiply Handicapped: The Choice is Yours. Governmental Affairs Dept. United Cerebral Palsy, Chester Arthur Bldg., 425 I Street, N.W., Washington, D.C. 20001 (selected papers).

Dickman, Irving R. *No Place Like Home: Alternative Living Arrangements for Teenagers and Adults with Cerebral Palsy.* United Cerebral Palsy, 66 E. 34th Street, New York, New York 10016 ($2.25).

Gini, Laurie. *Housing and Home Services for the Disabled.* Hagerstown, Maryland: Harper & Row ($20.00).

Housing for the Handicapped and Disabled. National Association of Housing & Redevelopment Offices, 2600 Virginia Avenue, N.W., Suite 404, Washington, D.C. 20037 (Publication # N588, $6.50).

HUD Programs That Can Help the Handicapped (brochure). Office of Independent Living, Department of Housing and Urban Development, Washington, D.C. 20410.

Pieper, Betty. Beyond the Family and the Institution: Residential Issues for Today (booklet). Spina Bifida Association of America, 343 S. Dearborn, Chicago, Illinois 60604 ($1.00).

RECREATION

Annand, Douglas. *The Wheel Chair Traveler.* Douglas R. Annand: Ball Hill Road, Milford, New Hampshire 03055.

Easter Seal Directory of Resident Camps for Persons with Special Help Needs. National Easter Seal Society for Crippled Children and Adults, 2023 W. Ogden Avenue, Chicago, Illinois 60612 ($1.50).

International Directory of Access Guides. Rehabilitation World, 20 W. 40th Street, New York, New York 10018.

List of Guidebooks for Handicapped Travelers. President's Committee on Employment of the Handicapped, Washington, D.C.

National Parks and Campgrounds. U.S. Forest Service, 633 W. Wisconsin Avenue, Milwaukee, Wisconsin 53203.

National Park Guide for the Handicapped. U.S. Government Printing Office, Washington, D.C.

Reamy, Lois. *Travel Ability: A Guide for Physically Disabled Travelers in the United States.* New York: MacMillan Publishing Co. ($9.95).

Travel Tips for the Handicapped. Consumer Information, U.S. Travel Service, U.S. Department of Commerce, Washington, D.C. 20230.

SEX

Berman, Sue. *Sexuality and the Spinal Cord Injured Woman.* Sister Kenny Institute, Publications Office, Dept 191, 1800 Chicago Avenue, Minneapolis, Minnesota 55404.

Gordon, Sol. *Sexual Rights for People . . . Who Happen to Be Handicapped.* Center on Human Policy, 216 Ostrom Avenue, Syracuse, New York, 1974.

The Handicapped and Sexual Health. SIECUS Report. ED-U Press, 760 Ostrom Avenue, Syracuse, New York.

Marriage and Parenting: Issues for People with Disabilities and Their Parents. Reprints # S-75. Exceptional Parent Bookstore, 296 Boylston Street, Boston, Massachusetts 02116 ($2.50).

Mooney, Thomas; Cole, Theodore and Chilgren, Richard. *Sexual Options for Paraplegics and Quadriplegics.* Boston: Little, Brown & Co., 1975.

TOYS AND PLAY

Buist, C. A. and Schulman, J. L. *Toys and Games for Educationally Handicapped Children.* Springfield, Illinois: Charles C. Thomas, 1976.

Carlson, B. W. and Ginglend, D. R. *Play Activities for the Retarded Child.* Nashville: Abingdon Press, 1961.

Karnes, Merle B. *Creative Games for Learning: Games for Parents and Children to Make.* Council for Exceptional Children, Publication Sales, 1920 Association Drive, Reston, Virginia 22091 ($7.50).

Physical Activities for the Mentally Retarded: Ideas for Instruction. American Alliance for Health, Physical Education and Recreation, 1201 16th Street, N.W., Washington, D.C. 20036.

Stepping Stones: Toys to Share with Handicapped Children. The State University of New York, 55 Elk Street, Albany, New York 12234, 1976.

INDEX